Encyclopedia of Cupping Therapy

(Al-Hijama)

I0483832

By

Izharul H. MD (PSM)

Rajiv Gandhi University, Bangalore

India

CSI Publishing Platform, South Carolina,
North Charleston, USA

Book Details

Paperback: 182 pages
Publisher: CSI Publishing Platform; 2 edition (March 2015)
Language: English
ISBN-10: 1508981507
ISBN-13: 978-1508981503
Product Dimensions: 6 x 9 inches

@**2014-15** by publishing platform and author

Corresponding email: drizharnium@gmail.com

Contact: 91-8287833547
Encyclopedia of cupping therapy
First Edition: 2014
Second Edition 2015
Publisher: CSI Publishing Platform; 2nd edition

ACKNOWLEDGEMENT

First and foremost, I have to thank my parents for their love and support throughout my life. Thank you both for giving me strength to reach the stars and chase my dreams. My brothers, sisters, and other family members deserve my wholehearted thanks as well.

I would like to express my gratitude to the many people who saw me through this book; to all those who provided support, talked things over, read, wrote, offered comments, allowed me to quote their remarks and assisted in the editing, proofreading and design.

I would like to thank my wife for standing beside me throughout my career and writing this book. She has been my inspiration and motivation for continuing to improve my knowledge and move my career forward.

I would like to thanks my all friends for understanding and encouragement in my many, many moments of crisis. Your friendship makes my life a wonderful experience. I cannot list all the names here, but you are always on my mind.

I wish to express my solemn sentiments and sincere gratitude to all the authors and researches of various textbooks and journal articles which was referred to, while preparing the manuscript of the book without which the scientific base of facts mentioned would not have been possible.

Once again thanks my parents and family members, for sharing my happiness when starting this book and following with encouragement when it seemed too difficult to be completed. I would have probably given up without their support and example on what to do when you really want something.

Last but not least, I wish to offer my apologies to all my colleagues and friends whose name has been omitted inadvertently, for without their constant support, encouragement and well-wishes, the book would not have been completed.

Thank you, Lord, for always being there for me.

Izharul H.

About the Author

Dr. Izharul H is a Registered Medical Doctor of Traditional alternative Medicine focused on general alternative medicine/Unani medicine family practice using the natural, holistic system of Traditional Unani Medicine.

His main goal is to nurture vibrant health in partnership with clients through safe, effective use of the following Unani medicine/regimenal/therapies:

- ❖ Cupping (including Wet Cupping or Hijama and Fire cupping)
- ❖ Acupuncture & Moxibustion
- ❖ Unani Herbal Medicine & Diet
- ❖ Medical Massage/Ayurvedic and Unani massage
- ❖ Leech therapy
- ❖ Vein section

His treatments are uniquely effective in acute pain relief, detoxifying of the body, Lipid profile management, hypertension, heart problems, and boosting immunity and circulation through combinations of WET cupping, acupuncture and/or herbal Unani medicine.

Skills:

- ❖ High lipid profile management
- ❖ Hypertension managmement
- ❖ Coronary Heart diseases management by Cupping therapy
- ❖ Migraine treatment
- ❖ Sexual diseases like sexual weakness, premature ejaculation

❖ Women's diseases, gynecological problems management
❖ Detoxification of body through cupping therapy
❖ Acute/Chronic pain management/Fibromyalgia

Qualifications

1. Bacheolar of Unani medicine and surgery (BUMS), Kanpur University, Kanpur India
2. Doctor of Medicine (MD), Rajiv Gandhi University, Bangalore, Karnataka, India
3. Clinical intern Govt district hospital, Allahabad, India
4. Assisstant proff, Dept of Juris & Toxi, Delhi University, Delhi, India
5. Registration Bhartiya chikitsa parisad

Certificates awarded:

1. **Perspectives in Rheumatology: Emerging Approaches to Management** by Medical Education Resources, Inc. 1500 West Canal Court Bldg B Littleton, CO 80120-6404.
2. **CME REPORT: New Frontiers in Type 2 Diabetes Mellitus Management: Introducing the Role of the Kidney as a Therapeutic Target** by NEW JERSEY ACADEMY OF FAMILY PHYSICIANS 224 West State Street Trenton, New Jersey 08608.
3. **COPD and Asthma: Addressing the Challenges of Differential Diagnosis and Treatment** by Medical Education Resources, Inc. 1500 West Canal Court Bldg B Littleton, CO 80120-6404.
4. **HIV/AIDS - Awareness & Prevention** by Alison Certificate Number: 268-674878.
5. **Modern Lifestyle Diseases: Awareness and Prevention** by Alison Certificate Number: AC-355-674878.

6. CME **"Life style medicine: Nutrition and the metabolic syndrome"** by THE Harvard Medical School.
7. CME **"Challenging cases in toxicology"** by THE Harvard Medical School.
8. **"Fundamentals of Sample Preparation Used in Toxicology"** by American Association for Clinical Chemistry, Washington.

Dr Izharul Hasan
Sultanpur Kunhari
District Haridwar
Uttarakhand
247663
Email: drizharnium@gmail.com
(M) 91-8287833547

About the book

For over 5,000 years, cupping has been used across the globe to treat a broad spectrum of health disorders. A safe, comfortable therapy, it requires only simple, inexpensive instruments to achieve highly effective results. This comprehensive book features all the information practitioners need, including historical facts, step-by-step instructions for application and treatment of specific health problems.

Cupping is a technique where glass, plastic, bamboo, or rubber cups are attached to the skin by negative pressure. The vacuum is generally used to pull out external influences that have invaded the body (heat, cold, dampness, wind) and are causing pain or illness. Cups are also used to support tired, overused or injured tissue assisting in rejuvenation and healing.

Encyclopedia of Cupping Therapy describes the history, methods and techniques of cupping therapy and provides practical guidelines for cupping therapy home use and professional practice. It provides a new classification of cupping therapy types and uses a new classification of cupping therapy points. It looks closely at issues of mechanism of action, side effects, treatment programs and safety.

Exploring the role of cupping therapy in a variety of clinical contexts which range from the treatment of children to the effective management of sports injuries and myofascial pain this well-established, highly successful book retains its useful step-by-step approach to the effective application of traditional cupping techniques with special emphasis on issues of safety, expectation and theoretical principles of action.

Encyclopedia of Cupping Therapy contains many of clear illustrations and provides a practical guideline for treating many of common diseases. Encyclopedia of Cupping Therapy includes new scientific researches and clinical examples. This book can serve as a useful reference for complementary and alternative medicine therapists, medical physicians, medical students, healthcare professionals and people interested in self-care and treatment. Actually the book puts in the hands of the readers the true Cupping method and helps them to differentiate between the true Cupping and the other false method of applying Cupping.

This text is the most complete and up to date book on cupping therapy (*Hijamah*) at this time, it cuts straight into the subject and quenches the curiosity of the reader whether it be a layperson, prospective patient or seasoned medical professional. Dr Izhar's experience and insight into Hijamah and traditional medicine as well as his strictness in correlating it with scientific findings is reflected throughout this guide. The author shares with you the complete and comprehensive depth to this topic and empowers the reader in understanding and applying the concepts, rules and guidelines regarding Hijamah in order to improve general health and benefit from this oft misunderstood and sometimes feared medical procedure.

The importance of this book is clear in establishing and clarifying the true method of practising Cupping therapy and in manifesting the scientific precise rules of true scientific hygienic Cupping. These rules control the Cupping procedure therefore they prevent any side effect and make it very fruitful.

The book Encyclopedia of cupping therapy shows the high effectiveness of true cupping in curing the incurable diseases and chronic ones. You read in this book the scientific explanation of each of the rules which control Cupping procedure, Cupping and its site from person's body, Cupping and physiological conditions of human body, and between Cupping and having food. In addition, you read in this book very important scientific notes and advices, and you notice the true Cupping operation step by step. Actually the main book of true Cupping from which this book is quoted is considered the first precise scientific reference of true cupping.

This edition is complete guide to cupping therapy book. This book is a complete cupping therapy professional lessons, to help to understand cupping therapy and how to use this effective therapy for various diseases. It is an illustrated book for complementary and alternative medicine professionals, students and supporters.

Dr Izharul Hasan

Sultanpur Kunhari

District Haridwar

Uttarakhand, 247663

Email: drizharnium@gmail.com

(M) 91-8287833547

"If we all treat each other like we treat ourselves- what a wonderful place earth would be."

INDEX

SN	Chapter	Page
1	Cupping Therapy/Al-Hijama	15-18
2	History of Cupping Therapy	19-31
3	History of Chinese Medicine Cupping	32-42
4	Cupping Therapy in Islam	43-45
5	The Precise Scientific Medical Rules for Cupping Therapy	46-61
6	Traditions About Cupping Therapy	62-66
7	Types of Cupping and Indications	67-76
8	Mechanism and Theories About How Cupping Therapy Works	77-104
9	Indications of Cupping Points/Places for Various Diseases	105-127
10	Clinical Researches done on Cupping Therapy	128-137
11	Safety, Preliminaries, Process, Precautions, and Contraindications of Cupping	138-147
12	Frequently Asked Questions (FAQs)	148-156
13	Patients Information	157-159
14	Few Clinical Cases Pictures for Demonstration	160-173
15	Summary and References	174-182

Chapter 1

CUPPING THERAPY/AL-HIJAMA

CUPPING THERAPY/AL-HIJAMA

The word "cupping" is derived from the Arabic verbs "Hajama" and "Haj'jama" which they mean "to minimize" or "to restore to basic size", or "to diminish in volume".

In Arabic they say, "A certain person diminished the problem", they meant that he returned the problem to its original size. There is also a verb "ahjama" which means "to withdraw or retreat from attack". Thus he who performed the cupping therapy made diseases refrain from attacking him. The increase of spoiled blood in the body rendered its cessation from growing when the person became twenty-two years old, and it accumulated in the back area of the person. With advance in age, these accumulations of spoiled blood hindered the circulation of the whole blood, eventually paralyzed the work of the young red corpuscles then the body became weak and exposed to various kinds of diseases. When one performed cupping, the blood returned to its original condition and the stagnant blood went away (that blood which contained maximum rate of senile red corpuscles and their cells ghosts and abnormal shapes of red blood cells, and other impurities).

It is an ancient medical treatment that relies upon creating a local suction to mobilise blood flow in order to promote healing. There are two types of Cupping Therapy (CT); Dry Cupping and Wet Cupping Therapy. In Dry Cupping, cups are placed on the skin for a period of with suction causing localized hyperaemia and healing is encouaraged. In Wet Cupping however, cups with suction are placed on the skin for a couple of minutes followed by superficial skin incision being made to the cupped skin. A small quantity of blood is then extracted from the skin. The blood extracted is believed to be harmful to the body and its removal brings about relief and healing.

Cupping is an ancient method of treatment that has been used in the treatment and cure of a broad range of conditions throughout the Eastern and Western cultures of the world. Conditions such as blood related disorders; haemophilia and hypertension for example, rheumatic conditions ranging from arthritis, sciatica, back pain and migraines through to psycho-social applications in the treatment of anxiety and general physical and mental well-being. Traditional theories advocate that the primary aim of Cupping is to extract blood that is believed to be harmful from the body which in turn rids the body of potential harm from symptoms leading to a reduction in well-being. To date there are no scientifically approved research trials anywhere in the world which investigated the impact of Cupping at a physiological level, although numerous small scale studies have been done promoting the benefits of Cupping for various diseases.

Cupping Therapy, commonly referred to as Cupping, has been around for thousands of years. It developed over time from the original use of hollowed out animal horns (the Horn Method) to treat boils and suck out the toxins out of snakebites and skin lesions. Horns slowly evolved into bamboo cups, which were eventually replaced by glass. Therapeutic applications evolved with the refinement of the cup itself, and with the cultures that employed cupping as a health care technique.

Chapter 2

HISTORY OF CUPPING THERAPY

HISTORY OF CUPPING THERAPY

The use of Cupping Therapy is documented in the history of most great cultures and civilizations of the past with the earliest available records revealing extensive use by the ancient Egyptians, Chinese and Middle Eastern cultures. Hippocrates (400 BC) is known to have written in detail about Cupping Therapy. The *Ebers Papyrus* (1550 BC), the oldest known medical text, also contains information on this subject.

The true origin of cupping still remains uncertain to this day. Some consider the Chinese to be responsible for cupping, however, the earliest pictorial records date back to the ancient Egyptians around 1500 B.C. Translations of hieroglyphics in the Ebers Papyrus, the oldest medical text book, detail the use of cupping for treating fever, pain, vertigo, menstrual imbalances, weakened appetite and helping to accelerate the healing crisis.

From the Egyptians, cupping was introduced to the ancient Greeks, where Hippocrates, the Father of Modern Medicine and cupping advocate, viewed cupping as a remedy for almost every type of disease. In fact, other Greek physicians used the strong suction of cupping to restore spinal alignment by reducing dislocated vertebrae from protruding inward.

The earliest recorded use of cupping came from the famous alchemist and herbalist, Ge Hong (281-341 A.D.), who popularized the saying "Acupuncture and cupping, more than half of the ills cured."

The Chinese expanded the utilization of cupping to include its use in surgery to divert blood flow from the surgery site. In the 1950's, after much extensive research, a collaborative effort between the former Soviet Union and China confirmed the clinical efficacy of cupping therapy. Since then, cupping has become a mainstay of government-sponsored hospitals of Traditional Chinese medicine.

Eventually, cupping spread to ancient cultures in many countries of Europe and even the Americas. Throughout the 18th century, European and American doctors widely used cupping in their practices to treat common colds and chest infections, often in the form of Wet Cupping. Wet Cupping, also known as Artificial Leeching and Hijamah in Muslim societies, is where the practitioner makes tiny incisions in the skin to dredge the blood or poisons out.

By the late 1800's, cupping lessened in popularity and was severely criticized and discredited by the newly established scientific model of medicine. The new model defined medicine by making the body transparent, focusing on and treating the inside, in preference to the outside. Since cupping was a surface treatment, it was inconsistent with this new medical paradigm, which had shifted away from hands-on manipulative therapies.

Decades flew by as cupping therapy gradually became reduced to a mere curiosity of the past, collecting dust on practitioners' shelves. In 2004 Cupping re-emerged as a hot new celebrity trend in the lime light of a New York film festival, where actress Gwyneth Paltrow's back revealed her fresh cupping marks. Countless celebrities like Jennifer Aniston, Victoria Beckham and Denise Richards followed suit and became fast adopters of this hot new cupping trend. Unfortunately, some of the Hollywood buzz viewed the celeb's cupping marks as simply bruises and rolled their eyes at its potential benefits.

Until recently, there was scant published evidence in favor of cupping for pain relief. Over the past three years however, a handful of new studies have shown it helps relieve back, neck, carpal tunnel and knee pain. One thing is certain, and that is cupping is a powerful healing modality that can complement many healthcare modalities ranging from spa treatments to medical massage and physical therapy.

Cupping Therapy is also referred by its local names; Hijamah in the Middle East and hacamat in Turkish cultures. In the west, Cupping Therapy was part of the basic repertoire of clinical skills a doctor would be expected to understand and practice until the latter part of the Nineteenth Century with some Eastern European countries such as the Balkans and Bulgaria continuing to practice Cupping Therapy to this very day.

The practice virtually disappeared from western medical cultures in the 20th Century however the Middle East, Chinese and Turkish cultures were able to preserve this technique in its natural form whilst adhering to safe current medical practice. In Chinese cultures because it conforms to the chi-theory of healing and in the Islamic World as it received religious encouragement by the Prophet Mohammed (pbuh).

In parts of Western Europe there has been a recent upsurge in the interest from both public and academic perspectives. Scientific studies have began researching the effects of Cupping Therapy in an attempt to better understand the mechanisms underpinning this fascinating medical treatment that has truly withstood the test of time. Celebrity endorsements by Professional sports players (Football Players and Olympic Swimmers) through to leading

Hollywood actresses have further raised the profile of Cupping Therapy.

Some Chinese and American schools of medicine teach Cupping Therapy as part of their Complementary Medicine programs. In Germany and England, some Medicine and Health Sciences faculties provide Cupping Therapy as elective modules. Esteemed universities in Turkey are currently conducting Cupping Therapy based research. Currently, the Turkish Ministry of Health is overlooking applications of Cupping Therapy to ensure safety and high quality standards.

A BRIEF HISTORY OF CUPPING

By Bruce Bentley

Way back in time, long before any historical or archeological evidence had been uncovered to support the application of cupping instruments to the body as a therapeutic procedure, prehistoric humans relied in part on their ability to suck and draw to the surface any irritations such as stings and thorns. Early humans also developed conceptualizations concerning their place in nature and the universe and the causes of ill health.

In their efforts to explain sickness, they held beliefs about that which could enter the body or mind such as evil spirits and cause pain and suffering. Many researchers including anthropologists have described how healers of these super naturalistic traditions of illness causation applied oral suction to the surface of the body to withdraw the effects of these malevolent influences.

The Horn method cupping

In time, various natural resources began to be used to effect suction - which makes good sense because indigenous groups could exploit their natural resources. For example, natives along the west coast of North America, in the vicinity of Vancouver Island, used shells. In Europe, Asia, Africa and North America, hollow animal horns were fashioned to provide an effective cupping device. In North America, the natives made their cupping implements by slicing off the point of a buffalo horn. They would then place the base of the horn on the body and suck the air out through the opening at the tip. When a vacuum was achieved, a wad of dried grass would be immediately thrust into the opening by the nimble workings of the tongue. By this method the medicine men, with their powerful facial muscles and considerable agility, can make a very succcssful job of cupping. (Brockbank, 1987:22). Another technique used to withdraw disease was by sucking through a bone tube. During the Babylon - Assyrian Empire (stretching from Iraq to the Mediterranean) massage was practised as well as 'cupping by sucking, with the mouth or by using a buffalo horn' (Mettler, 1947:320). The source of this information was presumably found inscribed on clay tablets, written in one of the earliest written languages, ie. cuneiform script around 700BC.

Hippocrates and the European traditions of cupping

Textual evidence on cupping can be found in thc writings of Hippocrates (C.460-377 BC), known as the Father of Modern Medicine. During this golden era of the early Greek state, Hippocrates and his followers were devoted to an empiric approach to healing and sought naturalistic explanations why people became ill. They thoroughly rejected causes like spirits or ghosts, and instead reasoned that poor diet, insufficient exercise, exposure to adverse weather, an unbalanced lifestyle and emotional factors were the chief agents of ill health. In his guide to clinical treatment, Hippocrates recommended cupping for the treatment of angina, menstrual irregularities and other disorders.

In the 1800's, the British cupper Samuel Bayfield (1839: 51-52), wrote: "Hippocrates was a minute observer, and has left us some striking remarks on the shape and application of the cups. He recommends that they should be small in diameter, conical in shape, and light in their weight, even when the disease for which they are applied is deeply seated".

Cupping refers to an ancient Chinese practice in which a cup is applied to the skin and the pressure in the cup is reduced (by using change in heat or by suctioning out air), so that the skin and superficial muscle layer is drawn into and held in the cup. In some cases, the cup may be moved while the suction of skin is active, causing a regional pulling of the skin and muscle (the technique is called gliding cupping).

This treatment has some relation to certain massage techniques, such as the rapid skin pinching along the back that is an important aspect of tuina (12). In that practice, the skin is pinched, sometimes at specific points (e.g., bladder meridian points), until a redness is generated. Cupping is applied by acupuncturists to certain acupuncture points, as well as to regions of the body that are affected by pain (where the pain is deeper than the tissues to be pulled). When the cups are moved along the surface of the skin, the treatment is somewhat like guasha (literally, sand scraping), a folk remedy of southeast Asia which is often carried out by scraping the skin with a coin or other object with the intention of breaking up stagnation. Movement of the cups is a gentler technique than guasha, as a lubricant allows the cup to slide without causing as much of the subcutaneous bruising that is an objective of guasha. Still, a certain amount of bruising is expected both from fixed position cupping (especially at the site of the cup rim) and with movement of the cups.

Traditional cupping, with use of heated cups, also has some similarity to moxibustion therapy. Heating of the cups was the method used to obtain suction: the hot air in the cups has a low density and, as the cups cool with the opening sealed by the skin, the pressure within the cups declines, sucking the skin into it. In this case, the cups are hot and have a stimulating effect something like that of burning moxa wool.

In some cases, a small amount of blood letting (luoci; vein pricking) is done first, using a pricking needle, and then the cup is applied over the site. The pricking is usually done with a three-edged needle, applied to a vein, and it typically draws 3-4 drops of blood (sometimes the skin on either side is squeezed to aid release of blood). A standard thick-gauge acupuncture needle or plum blossom needle may be used instead. This technique is said to promote blood circulation, remove stasis, and alleviate swelling and pain. It is employed especially when there is a toxic heat syndrome and for a variety of acute ailments.

The following report is derived mainly from a survey of reported cupping techniques published in 1989 (1), supplemented by information from acupuncture text books (5-9).

EARLY HISTORY

The earliest use of cupping that is recorded is from the famous Taoist alchemist and herbalist, Ge Hong (281-341 A.D.). The method was described in his book A Handbook of Prescriptions for Emergencies, in which the cups were actually animal horns, used for draining pustules. As a result of using horns, cupping has been known as jiaofa, or the horn technique. In a Tang Dynasty book, Necessities of a Frontier Official, cupping was prescribed for the treatment of pulmonary tuberculosis (or a similar disorder). More recently, Zhao Xuemin, during the Qing Dynasty, wrote Supplement to Outline of Materia Medica, including an entire chapter on "fire jar qi" (huoquan qi). In it, he emphasized the value of this treatment, using cups made of bamboo or pottery, in alleviating headache of wind-cold type, bi syndrome of wind origin, dizziness, and abdominal pain. The cups could be placed over acupuncture needles for these treatments. One of the traditional indications for cupping is dispelling cold in the channels. This indication is partly the result of applying hot cups. For example, bamboo cups would be boiled in an herbal decoction just prior to applying to the skin (this is one type of shuiguanfa, or liquid cupping, so-called because a liquid is incorporated into the treatment). Both liquid cupping and cupping over an acupuncture needle are favored for treatment of arthralgia. Cupping also is thought to dispel cold by virtue of its ability to release external pathogenic factors, including invasion of wind, damp, and cold.

Chapter 3

THE HISTORY OF CHINESE MEDICINE CUPPING

THE HISTORY OF CHINESE MEDICINE CUPPING

Chinese medicine uses many modalities of healing; acupuncture, herbal medicine, massage, and diet therapy make up the most commonly used and Chinese medicine cupping is gaining in popularity. Maybe some of you saw the photo a few years ago of Gwyneth Paltrow on the red carpet with a backless dress and cupping marks all up her spine? Sometimes it takes a little popular culture to remind us of ancient ways of healing!

The therapy of cupping has been used in China for thousands of years. At first it was applied using cattle horns or cross sections of bamboo. To create negative pressure inside the horn or bamboo these ancient 'cups' where boiled in water or fire was ignited to expel the air and suck the cups onto the skin. These cups were used mostly to draw out pus and blood in the treatment of boils. Cupping was originally used as an auxiliary method in traditional Chinese surgery. Later it was found to be useful in treating other diseases and developed into a special therapeutic method.

The earliest record of cupping is in the Bo Shu (an ancient book written on silk), which was discovered in a tomb of the Han Dynasty. Several other ancient texts mention Chinese medicine cupping. Several centuries later another famous medical classic, Su Sen Liang Fang, recorded an effective cure for chronic cough and the successful treatment of poisonous snake bites using cupping therapy.

Through several thousand years of accumulated clinical experience, the clinical applications of cupping have become increasingly wide. Now Chinese medicine cupping is used to treat arthritic symptoms, asthma, the common cold, chronic cough, indigestion problems and some skin conditions.

There is a saying in China: "Acupuncture and cupping, more than half of the ills cured." Zhao Xue Ming, a doctor practicing more than 200 years ago, compiled a book entitled Ben Cong Gang Mu She

Yi, in which he describes in detail the history and origin of different kinds of cupping and cup shapes, functions and applications.

In mainland China the development of cupping therapy has been rapid. In the 1950's the clinical efficacy of cupping was confirmed by the co-research of China and acupuncturists from the former Soviet Union, and was established as an official therapeutic practice in hospitals all over China.

Today, as more people (including Gwyneth) seek alternative therapies to deal with their health problems, the use of traditional Chinese medicine, including cupping is increasing. Much of the cupping equipment and methods used today are exactly the same as they were in ancient times. Some electronic or mechanized pumps have been invented, and suction cups introduced, but to a great extent the majority of people practicing cupping today still use horn, bamboo or glass cups. One reason that cupping techniques remain the same as in ancient times is due to the fact that, with the exception of a handful of acupuncture practitioners, cupping is generally practiced in rural area where no or very little modern medicine is available.

The Chinese expanded the utilization of cupping to include its use in surgery to divert blood flow from the surgery site. In the 1950's, after much extensive research, a collaborative effort between the former Soviet Union and China confirmed the clinical efficacy of cupping therapy. Since then, cupping has become a mainstay of government-sponsored hospitals of Traditional Chinese medicine.

Eventually, cupping spread to ancient cultures in many countries of Europe and even the Americas. Throughout the 18th century, European and American doctors widely used cupping in their practices to treat common colds and chest infections, often in the form of Wet Cupping. Wet Cupping, also known as Artificial Leeching and Hijamah in Muslim societies, is where the practitioner makes tiny incisions in the skin to dredge the blood or poisons out.

Cupping affects the flow of Qi and blood. It helps draw out and eliminate pathogenic factors such as wind, cold, damp and heat. Cupping also moves Qi and Blood and opens the pores of the skin, thus precipitating the removal of pathogens through the skin itself.

MODERN CUPPING

During the 20th century, new glass cups were developed (see Figure 1). Common drinking glasses have been used for this purpose, but thick glass cupping devices have also been produced and are preferred. The introduction of glass cups helped greatly, since the pottery cups broke very easily and the bamboo cups would deteriorate with repeated heating. Glass cups were easier to make than the brass or iron cups that were sometimes used as sturdy substitutes for the others; further, one could see the skin within the cup and evaluate the degree of response.

The glass cups are depressurized by providing some fire in the cup to heat up the air within just prior to placement. For example, hold a cotton ball dipped in alcohol with a pincer, ignite it, hold it in the cup, then rapidly apply to the skin; this is called shanhuofa (flash-fire cupping; see Figure 2).

Sometimes, a small amount alcohol is put in the cup and lit; this method is called dijiufa (alcohol-fire cupping).

At the end of the 20th century, another method of suction was developed in which a valve was constructed at the top of the jar and a small hand-operated pump is attached so that the practitioner could suction out air without relying on fire (thus avoiding some hazards and having greater control over the amount of suction). Both glass and plastic cups were developed, though the plastic ones are not very well suited to moving along the skin once in place, as the edges are not entirely smooth and the strength of the cups is limited. The modern name for cupping is baguanfa (suction cup therapy).

In order to allow easy movement of the glass cups along the skin, some oil is applied. Medicated massage oils (with extracts of herbs) are particularly useful for this purpose. Since the cups are applied at room temperature, the indication of removing cold from the channels is no longer as applicable, at least to stationary cups. There is some friction generated with moving cups, so that there is a small but significant amount of heat applied by that method, especially if a warming oil is used as lubricant.

Generally, the cup is left in place for about 10 minutes (typical range is 5-15 minutes). The skin becomes reddened due to the congestion of blood flow. The cup is removed by pressing the skin along side it to allow some outside air to leak into it, thus equalizing the pressure and releasing it. Some bruising along the site of the rim of the cup is expected.

Today, cupping is mainly recommended for the treatment of pain, gastro-intestinal disorders, lung diseases (especially chronic cough and asthma), and paralysis, though it can be used for other disorders as well. The areas of the body that are fleshy are preferred sites for cupping. Contraindications for cupping include: areas of skin that are inflamed; cases of high fever, convulsions or cramping, or easy bleeding (i.e., pathological level of low platelets); or the abdominal area or lower back during pregnancy. Movement of the cups is limited to fleshy areas: the movement should not cross bony ridges, such as the spine. Following are some of the recommended treatment sites for various disorders.

WOMEN AND THEIR PRACTICE OF CUPPING

Throughout European history, most of the population were treated by local lay practitioners who could charge less and be consulted more readily than physicians. Even more convenient was the availability of cupping as a therapy within the household. An important role that women have occupied in traditional societies has been the one who is skilled in the knowledge and application of a broad range of treatments and remedies. 'Cross cultural studies show that women and, in particular, female heads of households represent a major source of therapeutic assistance in many societies.' (Fineman, 1989:25). I have been informed by reliable sources that in living memory, cupping in Greece, Holland, Russia and Turkey was usually performed by women. In Vietnam, the lay and semi-professional cuppers I met were all women. In 11th century Europe from the writings of the masters we do know that there were a great many women physicians who were held in high esteem and greatly sought after by patients' (Cumston, 1987:217)

By the thirteenth century, however, those universities including medical studies in their curriculums, excluded women from study. Thereafter there is a notable absence of women in traditional medical histories, because they concentrated on documenting 'official medicine,' rather than the 'popular' medicine practised by the people. Despitc the fact that non-official medicine has been poorly represented, women have playcd a major role in health care delivery and have been more important than men in the use and continuity of cupping practice.

THE DECLINE OF CUPPING FROM THE MID TO LATE 1800S

By the mid to late 1800s, cupping was sharply criticised by the medical fraternity and had fallen away as a popular method. There are a number of complex issues relevant to why this happened - so I will present only a couple of reasons. Firstly, it was during this period that the newly established scientific model of medicine began discrediting all other previously established traditional therapies in order to gain medical dominance. Secondly, the 'clinical gaze' which Foucalt (1976) took to define medicine, made the body transparent and looked at and treated the inside in preference to the outside. Because cupping is a surface treatment, it was inconsistent with the new paradigm, which 'moved away fromt he personal contact of the manipulative and hands-on therapies of earlier times" (Thearl, 1990:124). to become fascinated with the deeper layers of the body.

Opposition to cupping was therefore not based on a lack of effectiveness, but because of its lack of "fit" with the growing interests and authority of the medical fraternity. Although cupping has remained popular in some areas of Europe, the 20th century has certainly seen it wane in Anglo-Saxon society. I think a major reason for this is due to the ideological effectiveness of medicine in winning virtual control over all matters related to health and illness. As part of this process, for example, with the Medical Registration Act of 1858, 'Parliament had achieved what the doctors never could - it had symbolically at least united the much-divided medical profession, by defining them over and against a common other, not to say enemy.' (Porter, 1987: 45).

This was relayed onto a set of social processes that stigmatised cupping and changed people's attitude to many traditional practices. For a time, cupping was reduced to the curiosity shelf of the past. However over the past couple of decades the tide has turned and people are rediscovering that some practices have plenty of merit, as well as reinstate their own ability for self-care.

Chapter 4

CUPPING THERAPY IN ISLAM

CUPPING THERAPY IN ISLAM

Cupping was old as history and it was a divine monistic norm explained by the venerated prophets and they recommended people to practice it. Al'lah's envoy "Muhammad" (Communication with Al'lah and Peace are through him) resuscitated the procedures of cupping after being forgotten for a long time. He directed its application according to its original healthy rules.

He was so virtuous in enacting cupping for Moslems and the whole world. But on the elapse of many centuries on the passing away of the Al'lah's envoy "Mohammed" (cpth), the rules of cupping were gradually forgotten due to negligence, dereliction and abstention until those rules were obliterated and lost.

There were certainly some sinful hands that put much lies in it and its basics until people abstained from using it and forgot it completely. It was true that few people practiced it, but unluckily they did not get use of it, or they did not get healthy benefit of it at all until people disclaimed it for they did not get its promising benefit.

People used to perform cupping in winter and summer, or after physical toil and fatigue, or after breakfast though it must be applied before on fast before breakfast. But eventually, the late humane savant, Mohammad Amin Sheikho revived the norm (Sunnah) in its precise rules which were mentioned in his book.

He revealed its rules and put them in their exact place on the human body for application. He also put forth the general secret of its healing mechanism which said "to rid one`s self of impure blood". He returned this medical therapeutic art to its effective scientific role and disclosed its rules and principles to his acquaintances, relatives and friends. In turn, they informed their acquaintances, relatives, friends and neighbors and all the people until it spread in many countries and even all people.

When people gained great healthy physical, psychological and feasible benefits, they increased in number in using it during the last years. They realized marvels in curing incurable diseases of the era as cancer, paralysis, angina pectoris, hemophilia, migraine, and the like.

In Arabic, Cupping Therapy is called Al-Hijamah. Literally, this means to absorb and pull, and for the body, or the hijm (what is sucked), to return to its natural state. The word hacamat is often used in Turkish when cupping is combined with bloodletting as Wet Cupping Therapy. The practice was revitalized by both the use and recommendation by the Pophet Mohammed (pbuh). In over 100narrations from the Prophet Mohammed (pbuh) have been cited in different collections of hadith (saying and actions of the Prophet Mohammed [pbuh]). As a result, cupping therapy has both survived and florusihed under Islamic culture and was key feature in medical practice during the enlightenment years of Averoes (Ibn Sina) et al., paving the way for the development of modern western medicine as we know it today.

Chapter 5

THE PRECISE SCIENTIFIC MEDICAL RULES FOR CUPPING THERAPY

THE PRECISE SCIENTIFIC MEDICAL RULES FOR CUPPING THERAPY

The Precise scientific medical rules, elucidated by the medical team has used in its scientific research work, can be summarized as follows:

First: The place of body for applying the cupping therapy.

Second: The suitable age for cupping

Third: Time of the cupping

Fourth: The physiological situation of the body.

First: The place of person's body for applying the cupping therapy:

It is: near the lower end of the shoulder blade (the scapula) in the two symmetric locations between the spine and the inside limit of the scapula.

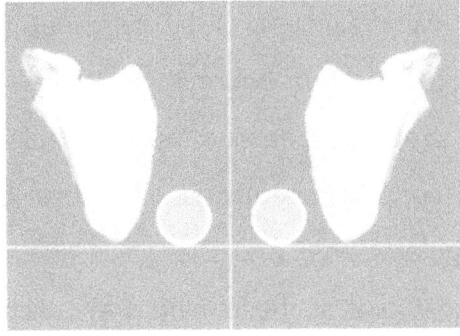

The cupping therapy makes a kind of blood congestion in the upper part of the back"these two symmetric places of back" by using (air cups). This cup is applied on the upper frontal part of the back, near the lower end of the scapulae and on the two sides of the spine.

This is because it is the calmest area in the body and void of moving joints. This area is a net of plexus capillaries of much ramification and profusion which makes the flow rate of blood circulation much less where the blood of the body precipitates its harmful precipitations (such as cell ghosts and dead of red blood cells) in it.

We made a lab study on this case, we found that the white corpuscles were less in this area of the back on the Cupping position other hand the cupping blood (the withdrawn blood by cupping) was full of cell ghosts, dead and abnormal red blood cells which made the cupping operation very suitable here. We per-formed cupping operations in places on the leg, the two jugular veins, and the back near the pelvis. The cupping blood in these places was similar to the vein blood.

Second: The suitable age for applying cupping therapy

Concerning men:

It is incumbent upon every male who reaches the twenty-two years of age to undergo cupping therapy from the seventeenth day of the lunar month which comes in the spring season of every year until the twenty-seventh day of it.

Childhood and adulthood stages require big quantities of iron because the body is in the phase of growth. These quantities are not completely supplied by food for this growing body. This decrease in iron is equalized by the way of digesting the senile and spoiled red blood cells in the liver and the spleen, and the phagocytes of the body forming the stored iron reserve which are kept for the body needs.

The body in general and its bone marrow in particular benefit from these red blood cells after transforming them suitably in a series of operations "metabolism" producing the iron (hemo) and amino acids (globin) which are used by the growing body to supply its need of iron in addition to reconstruction of new red generations of red blood cells .

After the twenty years, the big consumption of the spoiled red blood cells stops for the cessation of body's growth. So the surplus of them become big and "they must be discharged".

Concerning the women:

It is incumbent upon every female who passes the menopause stage. The woman has a natural outlet through which she can release herself from bad blood. During menstruation period, her blood circulation becomes at the apex of activity. When woman reaches her menopause stage, her menses ceases and she becomes subject to the same conditions of man who reaches the age of twenty-twenty two. Thus she enters a new physiological phase leading to psychological and physical changes paving the way to the rise of various diseases such as high blood pressure, coronary insufficiency and diabetes, and the like. In this situation, cupping becomes inevitable and there is no other alternative for it. It makes woman returns to her normal psychological and physical case. If she refuses to perform the simple cupping operation, her body becomes a pasture for maladies and prone to diseases.

Third: Timing of Applying Cupping therapy

To Apply Cupping you have to consider four appointed times:

1- The annual time:

The Messenger (cpth) said: "How good the wont in cupping is!"

Thus, it is usually performed from year to year for both the healthy and the patient. It is a prophylaxis for the healthy and a medicine (treatment) and a protection (prophylaxis) for the patient.

2- The seasonal time:

The Messenger (cpth) said, "Relieve yourselves from the intensity of heat by cupping."

Therefore cupping must be performed before the summer season because heat is most intense at this time of the year. Hence the best season is the spring. Cupping must be performed every year in the spring season, namely in April and May (In Syria and other countries around it).

Before giving the scientific interpretation of this appointed time (its physiological effect on our bodies), we must give a simple glimpse about the function of the blood in regulating the animal heat.

As it is known that water constitutes the maximum proportion in the blood, (90%) of its plasma. Since water has basic properties that differentiate it from other liquids known in nature, these properties make water the best assistant liquid to help regulating the animal heat in a living being. This property has a high faculty of storing heat than any other liquid or solid material. Therefore it stores the heat it receives in its passage through the more active and warm tissues and carries it to other tissues of less warmth in its movement through the various parts of the body.

Therefore blood has (the proportion of water in its formation and its round trip in the tissues of the body) a high faculty in transmitting heat higher than any other faculty of various tissues in the body. Therefore blood is the first recipient and the first main influenced tissue by the outside heat (of all the body tissues) which is effective on the body. It sucks heat from the body tissues to transport it to the less warm ones, and vice versa it sucks coolness from the body tissues to transport it to the warm ones.

In view of the continuous blood circulation, it acts in regulating the animal heat by warming the cool parts or cooling the warm parts until the animal heat remains constant. The chance for cupping is realized two times in the year, i.e. in April and in May, and perhaps a third time in late of March if the warmth comes at the end of it with only the decrease of the crescent.

In this time of the spring, we trace the lunar month until it becomes the 17th day of it, and then one can undergo cupping therapy in one of these days (from the seventeenth day until the twenty-seven day inclusive).

If he misses the first month, the advent of the (17th) of the next lunar month (in which cupping is permissible), he can also make up for the chance. Naturally, there are some irregular years when April is also intensive in chilliness, then we must wait until May, or we could perhaps perform the cupping therapy in April. If the (17) of the lunar month in April has cold weather, we wait until the weather becomes moderate and warm during the period of this lunar month (17-27) then we start cupping. Therefore, the matter is limited by the general rule which we cannot overcome for it is springtime (April, May and perhaps late of March and the early of June) from the seventeenth day until the twenty-seventh day of the lunar month exclusively depending on the rise in temperature in March and the drop of it at the beginning of June if both changes occur along with the decrease of the lunar month. In this way, we get use of one-third of the year to perform the cupping therapy.

3- The Monthly Time:

The Messenger of God (cpth) said, "Cupping is most detestable at the beginning of the crescent, but it is curing when the full moon begins to decrease."

Therefore, we must follow up the recommendation of the Messenger (cpth) on the lunar month when the time of the annual cupping comes (springtime in its two months, April and May).

For example, when April comes we follow up the progression of the lunar month which comes in this month (April), and when the seventeenth day of the lunar month comes, it will certainly be the first day for performing Cupping. Therefore, cupping starts from the seventeenth day (inclusive) until the twenty-seventh day (inclusive).

THE RELATION BETWEEN THE MOON AND CUPPING

What secret it was that made the Messenger (cpth) apprise of the time of cupping to be in the springtide with the progression of the lunar month from only the seventeenth day until the twenty-seventh day of it! We know that the moon has a pull effect on the earth despite its little diameter (3478 km), and its mass constitutes one part out of (80) parts of the mass of the earth, and the distance of it from the earth is a distance of (385.000 km), this short distance makes its pulling force have a great cupping starts from the seventeenth . day of lunar Month influence on the oceans where they rise to form the tide, even the earth's crust is never free from these effects.

The crust of the North American continent heaves up to fifteen centimeters when the moon interposes its sky. The moon has also another effect which helps sap to rise in its circulation in the high trees. The two French professors (Jubet and Galieh de Fond) noticed that the moon has an effect on animals from its birth as a crescent until it becomes a full-moon. The sexual activates increase gradually in animals, poultry and birds.

They also noticed that poultry give more eggs in thisvperiod more than the period of senility when the moonvbegins its gradual atrophy to hunchback phase, then to thevlast lunar quarter, and to waning. According to special notice, it is found that there is a period of activity and much energy in animals connected with the lunar stages. They also noticed that poultry and some domesticated animals, and

fishes, animals and lobsters of the Indian Ocean and the Red Sea produce more eggs in certain periods of the moon faces. The moon reaches the climax of its effect when it is fullmoon. It affects blood pressure producing higher level of pressure and in stimulating the blood circulation, so the sexual craving is excited. Also some western countries suffer much from the increase in the rate of crimes and assaults in nights and days of the full-moon.

During the first days of the lunar month, i.e. from the first day until of the fifteenth day, blood-flow is stimulated and it reaches its maximal limit and eventually it pokes all the blood residues and impurities which precipitated along the walls of the deep and superficial and in all the ramifications of the blood vessels in the tissues (exactly as, in turn, it - as a big spoon- stirs the water of the seas so as the salts in them don't precipitate). Likewise, when the moon begins to decrease from (17 - 27), the blood can carry these residues and impurities to the calmest parts of the body where they settle in the shoulder blades area.

The tide of the seas due to the lunar pull begins to weaken from 17 to 27 of the lunar calendar. Since the cupping therapy is performed in the morning after sleep and rest for the body and the blood circulation, and the moon is still rising despite the sunrise in the morning. The moon will have a little tidal effect during the performance of cupping. This situation is very good for our work for the moon still has the effect of pulling the blood from inside to the outside (the inner blood of the peripheral blood and the peripheral blood surrounding the opening of the cup). This situation has an excellent effect in performing a successful and profitable cupping therapy to release the body from its impure blood.

If the cupping therapy is performed in the middle of the lunar days (12-13-14-15), the strong pull of the moon stimulates the blood, and the blood will lose much of its young corpuscles, the Merciful God does not wish that for his servant-mankind. But the first days of the moon (crescent) do not let it do its job in carrying the blood residues and impurities from the inside to the outside in order to gather in the upper part of the back as it has been mentioned before.

4- The Daily Time:

The cupping therapy is usually performed in the early morning after the sunrise, but the time of stopping it in each day is pointed according to the heat level of the weather. If the weather stills moderate during the day, we continue applying it until noon; such timing is permissible but not desirable. It is better for cupping to be performed at the first hours of the day (because cupping must be performed while the person is still without having breakfast).

If a person remains without having breakfast for late hours of the day, he becomes tired and dizzy for the delay of having his breakfast and having performed the cupping therapy. In order to avoid all these problems and to perform a correct useful cupping operation, we must hasten to perform it in the early hours of the day from seven o'clock till ten o'clock, and in a needful situation when the time is the last day (27 of the lunar calendar) of performing it and the weather is still moderate and not intense in heat.

The cupping therapy is usually performed in the early morning after the sunrise this case you can perform the therapy until eleven o'clock or more before the noon. When we delay the therapy until (midday), we certainly walk, move and work. This motivates the blood circulation a little and scoops with it the harmful precipitations (such as cell ghosts and dead of red blood cells) which temporary precipitate under the shoulder blades, eventually the benefit from cupping is not complete.

Fourth: The Physiological Condition of the Body

The cupping therapy must be done before the breakfast. The Messenger of God (cpth) said, "Cupping before breakfast is optimal, and it has cure and benediction."

It is forbidden for a person to be cupped to take in any morsel whatsoever in the morning of cupping, but to remain fasting until it is performed upon him. He is permitted to drink a cup of coffee or tea for the sugar it contains is little and it does not need complicated digestive procedures which stir the blood, activate the blood circulation, affect the blood pressure, and the heart beats.

Also this little quantity of tea or coffee contains a simple nerve stimulant which makes the person undergo cupping in a wakeful case. For this reason the Prophet (cpth) prohibited eating before applying cupping for it activates the digestive system and the blood circulation in order to recompense the digestive operations which lead to the increase in heart beats, blood flow, and a high blood pressure. This case will move the precipitated residues of the sluggish and retired blood in the superficial and deep blood vessels and capillaries in the region of the upper back (these unwanted materials of blood gather during sleeping). Also blood flow is activated during the distribution of the digested nutrients in order to feed the body tissues. Such a situation does not fit cupping.

If cupping is performed in similar condition, the blood isn't filtered by this operation (Cupping), so the withdrawn blood is the working blood (not the spoiled blood which is full of impurities as dead red blood cells and R.B. cell ghosts) and we have lost the expected benefit from cupping. In this case, the cupped person will also suffer from slight vertigo or syncope as a result of the insufficient quantity of blood which irrigates the brain.

Chapter 6

TRADITIONS ABOUT CUPPING THERAPY

TRADITIONS ABOUT CUPPING THERAPY

As for those narrated traditions, which permit performing cupping on days of Monday, Tuesday and Thursday; and forbids its performance on days of Wednesday, Saturday and Sunday, were weakened by Alhafez Ibn Hijr in Alfat'h (the Conquest) (12/256), and the late Imam Almajlisi showed their contradictions. We shall, for exclusive example, bring a pattern for you and leave the verdict to you, my dear brother reader. The first tradition: From Ibn Omar "may God be pleased with him" said, "Apply cupping treatment on Thursday".

The second tradition: " Never be cupped on Thursday. He, who has been performed on, misfortune, affects him" .

Today, there are so many contradictory traditions which tell you to be cupped on Tuesday, and others tell you not to be cupped on such a day. This contradiction denotes to their falseness and incredibility, and aims at confusion and liquefaction of the traditions of the favorite Prophet about cupping. All these are prejudiced intrigues whereas the rightful one is the one which the clear logic accepts it through the practical fact, and that which you find it aligns with the tradition of the Messenger of God, that does not confine cupping on days of Saturday, or Sunday, or Monday, or Tuesday...etc. but it defines the cupping time according to the lunar month, from his saying: " Cupping is detested at the beginning of the crescent, and it is not hoped for benefit until the crescent decreases".

It was told by Al-Hindi in his Kanz Al-Ummal (28113), by al-Ajlouni in 'Kashf Al-khafa' (Uncovering of the concealment) , and by Ibn Al-Jawzi in Tathkarat Almawdhooaat /207/(Memo of subjects) .

This tradition was backed by another one in his saying: "The best days for you to be cupped are the seventeenth day, the nineteenth day, and the twentyfirst day (of the lunar month)"

This honored tradition denotes the incredibility of the traditions which prohibit most days of the week: Saturday, Sunday, Wednesday, Thursday, Friday, and Tuesday for a clear reason you yourself can discover it. Let us suppose that the seventeenth day of the lunar month comes on Friday and this means that the nineteenth day of it will surely be Sunday, and the twenty-first day of it will be Tuesday.

Let us also suppose that the seventeenth day comes on Thursday, then the nineteenth will be Saturday, and the twenty-first will be Monday... and so on. The inconstancy of the days in relation with the dates of the lunar month because the lunar month is changing from month to another, and from year to year.

This proves the abrogation of the traditions and of the claims that prohibit applying cupping on some days despite they are in a true time of performing cupping as they are in the spring time and after the decreasing of crescent, and it confirms the futility of such traditions in a clear way. The Prophet (cpth) is innocent of such fabrications.

Anas ibn Maalik (may Allaah be pleased with him) reported that the Messenger (Sallallaahu Álayhi Wasallam) said, **"Indeed the best of remedies you have is cupping (hijama)…"** [Saheeh al-Bukhaaree (5371)].

Abu Hurairah (may Allaah be pleased with him) reported that the Messenger (Sallallaahu Álayhi Wasallam) said, **"If there was something excellent to be used as a remedy then it is cupping (hijama)."** [Saheeh Sunan abi Dawud (3857), Saheeh Sunan ibn Maajah (3476)].

The Angels Recommending Cupping (Hijama)

Abdullah ibn Abbas (may Allaah be pleased with him) reported that the Messenger (Sallallaahu

Álayhi Wasallam) said, "I did not pass by an angel from the angels on the night journey except that they all said to me: Upon you is cupping (hijama), O Muhammad." [Saheeh Sunan ibn Maajah (3477)].

In the narration reported by Abdullah ibn Mas'ud (may Allaah be pleased with him) the angels said, "Oh Muhammad, order your Ummah (nation) with cupping (hijama)." [Saheeh Sunan Tirmidhee (3479)].

Chapter 7

TYPES OF CUPPING AND INDICATIONS

TYPES OF CUPPING

There are two main types of cupping:

Dry cupping: skin immediately below the cup is sucked up by a vacuum created inside the cup

Wet cupping: in which the skin immediately below the cup is cross cut superficially several times lightly lacerated; so that blood would actually be drawn out by the vacuum from the skin into the cup.

For both forms of cupping, the patient should be advised to increase their water intake.

Dry cupping is always used before wet cupping is considered. The use of whichever form of cupping is at the discretion of the practitioner.

OTHER METHODS OF CUPPING

In total there are 11 methods of cupping designed to help the practitioner choose the most appropriate cupping method for the patient. These methods are:

- ❖ Weak (light) cupping
- ❖ Medium cupping
- ❖ Strong cupping
- ❖ Moving cupping
- ❖ Light moving cupping
- ❖ Needle cupping
- ❖ Moxa (hot needle) cupping
- ❖ Empty (flash) cupping
- ❖ Full (bleeding/wet) cupping
- ❖ Herbal cupping
- ❖ Water cupping

Weak (light) Cupping

It is employed when blood and energy are sluggish or stagnant. The intention is move the stagnation and at the same time tonify the weak energy. The key factor in deciding when to apply weak cupping is the present energetic state of the patient. Evaluation of the pulse and tongue should all point to weakness. The amount of flesh drawn into the cup should be minimal and hardly raised. This method can be applied to almost anywhere on the body and may cause a slight reddening of the skin. Weak cupping is the most gentle method of all cupping and is particularly suitable for debilitated adults, elderly patients and young children, especially those under 7 years of age.

Medium cupping

This is the most frequently used method on patients. This method can safely be administered to children over 7 years of age. With medium cupping, suction is firmer pulling the skin well into the cup creating a slight redness. Medium cupping can safely be applied anywhere on the body.

Strong cupping

This is one of the most draining techniques. Therefore before deciding on this method, the practitioner must ensure the suitability of the patient. Pulse and tongue diagnosis should emphasize excess or fullness. This method may sometimes leave the patient feeling tired or drained. A strong vacuum need to be produced, giving a strong pulling sensation of the skin inside the cup. Because of the strong nature of the pulling action, the skin will quickly turn red and shortly turn purple inside the cup and possible erythema in the skin surrounding the cup. When using the strong cupping method for the first time, the mark is inevitable and can take 15-20 days to disappear completely. The cupping time should be short i.e. 5-10 minutes during the first session which can increase up to 20 minutes during later applications. **Strong cupping is often coupled with wet cupping**.

Moving cupping

The objective of this treatment is to apply strong cupping to a much larger area of the body by the moving/sliding action of the cup. This is the most painful cupping method and is often not practiced in Tibb.

Light moving cupping

Light moving cupping is practiced mainly on patients with relatively full/excessive energy. It is useful and considered the only safe method in the management of lymphatic drainage as well as being the exclusive cupping method in the management of cellulite complaints. During the application, slight pinkish cupping marks appear on the skin, normally following the direction and movement of the cup. At no time should deep, dark red cupping marks be seen. All cupping marks should fade away in a day or two. The whole objective of light cupping is to disperse stasis or stagnation without draining the patient. All moving cupping should require special attention particularly when the skin surface is broken, e.g. scratches, cuts, bruises, open wounds, etc.

Needle cupping and Moxa (hot needle) cupping

Not often practiced in Tibb as it follows acupuncture treatment. The cup is placed over the inserted acupuncture needle.

Empty (flash) cupping

Empty cupping is also called flash cupping for its speed during application. This is actually medium to strong cupping applied rapidly i.e. the cups remain in place for a very short period (<30 seconds). It is used to stimulate and move blood and energy in the weak and frail. The short duration is enough to stimulate physis and move blood but not enough to drain the patient. This can be repeated for between 5-10 minutes.

Full (bleeding/wet) cupping

This is the most favored and practiced method by practitioners. It is used in the treatment of a sudden increase in blood pressure, high fevers, blood stasis and in discharging pus from boils. This method is often combined with strong cupping. After the initial strong cupping, the cup is removed and slight superficial lacerations are made. The cup is then placed back on the site. Most of the blood in the cup will be semicoagulated and therefore still quite fluid. Before removing the cup, the practitioner should wear disposable surgical gloves on both hands.

Remove the cups gentle. It is not recommended to bleed the patient more than once a month and not to draw more than 100ml of blood at any one time.

Herbal cupping

For this method one requires a few bamboo cups, a relatively deep pan, water, metal clamps, some form of fire and herbs based in a prescription based on the treatment. The cups are boiled in the pan with water and the prescribed herbs. The cups are then placed on the patient in the traditional way using (Flame). The herbs are absorbed into the bamboo cups, which in turn transfer their healing properties to the patient. Cups can be left on for 10-20 minutes.

Precaution: following the boiling process, some steam remains inside the cup, resulting in a pressure build-up which pushes the cup away from the skin. This can be rectified by resting the hot bamboo cups on a dry towel for up to a minute in order to absorb excess water and at the same time reducing the pressure inside the cup.

Water cupping

This is one of the least used and practiced cupping methods. The technique involves filling a glass or bamboo cup one-third full with warm water and employing the cupping process quickly. Hold the cup close to the patient with one hand, bring it close to the point to be cupped and insert the burning cotton wool, swiftly and simultaneously turning the cup onto the skin. This method is said to disperse energy and resolve phlegm making it very beneficial for asthma, particularly in children. There is usually no mark left with this method.

How often can cupping be applied?

Children under the age of 16 - once a week is considered the acceptable frequency. Adults under the age of 60 - as much as twice a week (with the exception of wet cupping) Adults over the age of 70 - once a week However, during the 'acute stage' of a disease, treatment TDS or even once every day can be beneficial. Similarly, in all age groups when light, empty or light moving cupping is employed, treatment frequency can be increased to as much as once every other day. This is because blood, energy and the lymphatic fluids are gently stimulated rather than forcefully manipulated.

Indications:

* ❖ Blockages & Congestion
* ❖ Cholesterol & Uric Acid
* ❖ Hypertension
* ❖ Diabetes Control
* ❖ Gynecological Disorders
* ❖ Slip Disc, Sciatica
* ❖ Knee & all Joint pains
* ❖ Skin Conditions
* ❖ Severe Headaches
* ❖ Carpal Tunnel Syndrome
* ❖ Migraine
* ❖ Varicose Veins
* ❖ Upper & Lower Back Pain
* ❖ Obesity & Weight issues
* ❖ Arthritis & Rheumatism
* ❖ Frozen Shoulder & Neck
* ❖ Fatigue & Depression
* ❖ Anxiety & Stress

❖ Constipation & Diarrhea

❖ Asthma

❖ Cellulite

❖ Anemia

❖ Atrophy

❖ skin problems

❖ Common cold and flu

Chapter 8

MECHANISMS AND THEORIES ABOUT HOW CUPPING THERAPY WORKS

MECHANISMS AND THEORIES ABOUT HOW CUPPING THERAPY WORKS

Mode of action:

Cupping causes the tissues beneath the cup to be drawn up and swell, and an increase in blood flow to the affected area. This enhanced blood flow under the cup draws impurities and toxins away from the nearby tissues and organs to the skin, from where they are expelled. The release of the vacuum redirects "toxic" blood that had pooled at the site and redirects it to other areas of the body, thus allowing "fresh" blood to replace it. This facilitates the healing process. Localized and deep-tissue healing takes place. Cupping diverts toxins and impurities from important organs - such as the liver or kidney - to the less important organ, the skin. In dry cupping, the toxins are brought to the underlying skin; in wet cupping the toxins are brought out of the body, onto the surface of the skin.

The mechanisms of action of cupping therapy need to be elucidated. Many questions arise from time to time about the exact role of cupping in treating diseases and medical conditions that seem resistant to current treatment modalities. Many theories exist to explain benefits of cupping therapy. We will discuss briefly some of them to get a complete idea about how cupping therapy works.

Chinese theory for cupping therapy:

The concept and theory about mechanism of cupping therapy according to the Chinese theory need revision in light of modern medical scientific knowledge. Practitioners of cupping therapy in traditional Chinese medicine (TCM) may believe that diseases are caused by stagnation or blocking the source of vital energy of life (Qi). They believe that cupping therapy works by unblocking Qi and restoring correct balance to regain its flow . According to the traditional Chinese medical sexology, female gives Yin (female Qi) and receives Yang (male Qi), while male gives Yang and receives Yin. Both the Yin and Yang modalities of Qi are actively present in all males and females. It was explained that cupping therapy can remove the wind, cold, dampness and stagnant blood, especially when cupping therapy was combined with acupuncture. Laser acupuncture combined with cupping in the painful areas were thought to facilitate the flow of Qi in meridians according to Arndt-Schulz Biological Law.

Some scientists in the western world follow this theory e.g. Ilkay Chirali described ten methods of cupping therapy in his book entitled (Traditional Chinese Medicine Cupping Therapy). The ten cupping methods mentioned by the author included weak/light cupping, medium cupping, strong cupping, moving cupping, needle cupping, moxa/hot needle cupping, empty/flash cupping, full/bleeding cupping, herbal cupping and water cupping. The author mentioned some details about each type of cupping therapy and attributed the mechanisms of cupping therapy to be due to inducing changes in Qi (energy source), Xu (deficient blood), Wei Qi (defensive energy) and other concepts according to the Chinese theory. For example, fibromyalgia, in TCM, is mainly caused by emotional stress and depression, which affect the liver. Stagnation of Qi activity leads to stasis of blood that causes pain.

The principle of treatment is regulating the Qi and blood with dispelling cold and removing damp. However, the concepts of energy source and stagnant or deficient blood seem not to be in line with the basic scientific medical concepts. To discuss that from the medical and scientific point of view, it is worth saying that the source of energy in living cells come mainly from mitochondrial oxidative phosphorylation reactions in all body cells containing mitochondria. Added to that, glucose oxidation (glycolysis) is a cytoplasmic source of energy in body cells and its importance increases in cells lacking mitochondria as red blood cells (RBCs) and in cells having few numbers of mitochondria as neutrophils . Fatty acid oxidation and ketone bodies oxidation are other mitochondrial sources of energy. Energy production in mitochondria in cancer cells does not follow this rule as cancer cells are having mitochondrial mutations and are characterized by glycolytic phenotype in getting energy. Catabolism of glucose in cancer cells provides most of their energy source (ATP) and ends with production of lactate (Warburg effect) that is extruded outside cells. In previous publications by El Sayed et al., targeting energy glycolytic pathways selectively killed cancer cells and spared normal cells. Energy sources in cells do not seem to have any relation with cupping therapy. No scientific reports mentioned that cupping therapy can affect glycolysis or mitochondrial pathways for energy production.

Mechanisms of cupping therapy according to Hong et al:

Hong et al. reported that cupping therapy works via creating specific changes in local tissue structures as a result of local negative pressure in the cups used which stretches the nerve and muscle causing an increase in blood circulation and causing autohemolysis . When investigating the mechanisms proposed by Hong et al., it may be accepted to mention that local negative pressure may affect tissue structure and increase blood circulation but this is not enough to explain benefits of cupping therapy in treating cellulitis, migraine, headache, hypertension, CTS and others.

In addition to that, is autohemolysis beneficial for therapeutic benefit in previously mentioned diseases? The answer is negative. Hong mechanisms partially succeeded in explaining therapeutic effect of cupping therapy.

Mechanisms of cupping therapy according to Gao et al:

Gao et al. suggested that putting cups on selected acupoints on the skin produces hyperemia or hemostasis which results in a therapeutic effect. However, this seems not enough to explain therapeutic benefits of cupping therapy as regard effect of cupping therapy in treating RA, CTS, cellulitis and others.

Reported mechanisms for analgesic effects of cupping therapy:

Many possible mechanisms were reported to explain cupping induced analgesia when wet cupping therapy

(WCT) was used in treatment of CTS. Cupping therapy may induce deformation or injury to the skin leading to stimulation of β fibers in the painful region and distal skin regions and stimulation of inhibitory receptive fields of the multi-receptive dorsal horn neurons at the level of the spinal cord. In addition, cupping therapy may simulate special naturopathic setting leading to relaxation and comfort of the patient.

Cupping therapy induced analgesia may be similar to the effect of acupuncture and occurs via segmental, extra-segmental and central regulatory action. However, acupuncture differs from WCT as regard their mechanisms of action. Moreover, cupping induced skin laceration creates a vacuum on the skin and draws out a small amount of blood. Local damage of the skin and capillary vessels (induced by cupping) may cause a nociceptive stimulus that stimulates diffuse noxious inhibitory control in addition to the affective component of chronic musculoskeletal pain, which may relieve pain associated with the affective component through the limbic response.

Therefore, the tactile stimulus of cupping may be responsible for the analgesic effect. Cupping therapy enhances blood circulation, treats congestion and stops the inflammatory extravasations (escaping of some body fluids e.g. blood) from the tissues. Cupping may affect the autonomic nervous system and help to reduce pain. However, although previously mentioned explanations may explain analgesic effect of cupping therapy, it is still not enough to explain how cupping therapy itself treats so many diseases with different etiologies and pathogeneses.

Taibah theory (by Salah M. El Sayed) for scientific mechanisms of cupping therapy e.g. Al-hijamah (Cupping therapy of prophetic medicine):

Human body is kept under physiological homeostasis by the harmony of body systems and organs. Disease etiopathogenesis occurs against physiological homeostasis. Disease pathophysiology varies according to the etiology of each disease and its effect on disturbing body homeostasis. The beauty of cupping therapy comes from the fact that cupping therapy is an excretory form of therapy not an introductory one in which cupping removes blood and tissue fluids mixed with potentially harmful substances. We report here a novel simple theory to explain scientific mechanisms that govern the process and therapeutic benefits of cupping. Cupping seems to be related in principle to the scientific principles governing excretory functions of the kidney to the extent that cupping may be regarded as an artificial kidney that performs skin capillary filtration and size-dependent excretion of particles at pressures higher than filtration pressures in renal glomeruli.

While excretion through kidney is limited to hydrophilic materials, cupping therapy can excrete hydrophilic and hydrophobic materials as lipoproteins and enhance the natural excretory role of the skin.

Treatment using cupping therapy keeps human body away from a long list of undesired side effects and possible drug-drug interactions of therapeutic drugs. Searching for scientific principles of cupping urged us to propose a new mechanism to explain scientific and medical bases of cupping therapy, Taibah theory.

As cupping includes both dry cupping therapy and skin puncturing, first part of Taibah theory gives scientific principles of dry cupping therapy.

Taibah theory states that: Al-hijamah is wet cupping therapy of prophetic medicine (Arabic in origin). Al-hijamah includes all steps (and consequently similar or better therapeutic benefits) of both Chinese dry cupping therapy and wet cupping therapy altogether. Al-hijamah is related in principle to the scientific mechanisms underlying abscess evacuation and fluid filtration at renal glomeruli, where a pressure-dependent excretion of harmful substances and CPS occurs. CPS include both disease-causing substances and disease-related substances resulting during disease pathogenesis.

Al-hijamah is a minor surgical excretory procedure, where negative pressure (suction force) applied to skin surface using cups creates skin upliftings (gradually increasing in size due to viscoelastic nature of the skin) inside which local pressure correspondingly decreases (Boyle's law) around capillaries. This causes increased capillary filtration, local collection of filtered fluids, lymph and interstitial fluids and their retention inside skin uplifting. This dilutes chemical substances, inflammatory mediators, nociceptive substances, bathes nerve endings in collected fluids and breaks tissue adhesions causing decreased pain (Taibah theory for dry cupping therapy). On removing the cups, dramatic increase in skin blood flow occurs (reactive hyperemia).

Salah's theory for wet cupping therapy (WCT)is named Taibah theory (named after Taibah city, Al-Madinah Al-Munawwarah, city of Prophet Mohammad peace be upon him). In light of Taibah theory, prophetic method of WCT (Al-hijamah) can be defined as a minor surgical excretory procedure that creates superficial skin scarifications to open skin barrier and create a pressure gradient and a traction force across the skin and underlying capillaries to drain interstitial fluids and enhance blood clearance and waste excretion through skin. From Taibah theory, it can be concluded that WCT works through inducing local fluid collection in skin upliftings that comes out through inducing skin scarifications leading to decreased interstitial fluid pressure and clearance of interstitial spaces. This causes a pressure gradient and traction force across the walls of blood and lymphatic capillaries in the cupped area to drain solutes and fluids to interstitial spaces then through skin scarifications to outside. This enhances blood circulation and lymph flow and directs filtered fluids (including lymph) to the cupped area with further clearance of blood and lymph in the short time period during which negative suction is applied. This may help to regain homeostasis in human body.

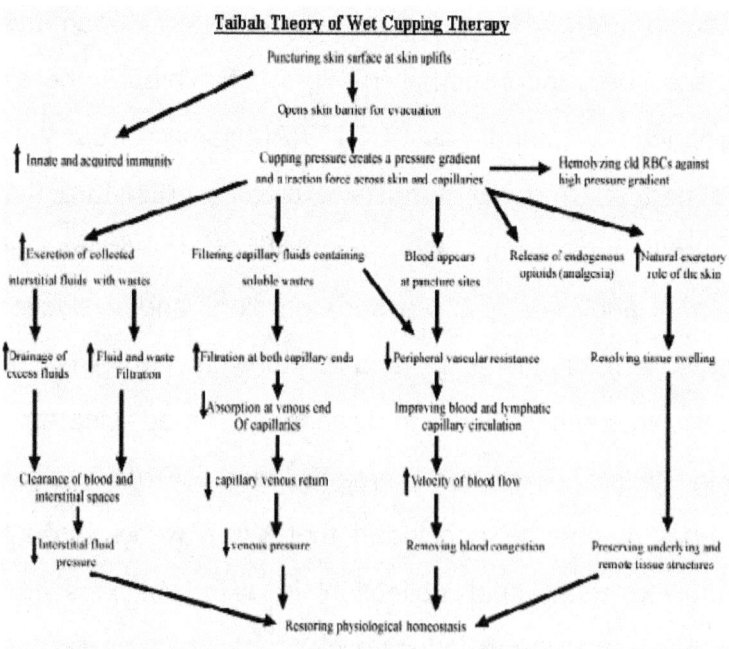

Taibah Theory of Wet Cupping Therapy

Medical Perspective in Understanding Some Mechanisms Followed by the Cupping therapy to Cure or Improve a number of Hopeless Diseases

Role that cupping may play in spleen diseases:

Splenomegalies may be due to the need of increasing the splenic work. For example, some reasons which causes these Splenomegalies are; Infectious inflammatory causes: It is believed that this kind of Splenomegaly caused by infectious inflammatory factor results from the increasing in spleen's defensive activity, or due to the increasing need to refine certain compounds from the blood.

And the congestive causes: this kind of Splenomegaly caused by the congestive causes results from the increase in pressure in portal circulation or in the general blood circulation. The amplification may also be due to over productivity of reticals-endothelia cells for the spleen to withdraw the spoiled cells from the blood, or due to the myeloid metaplasia, or the amplification may be due to blood rubeosis, or infiltration lesion where the spleenphagias are filled with spoiled materials which accumulated due to the effect of these diseases.

We have found in this respect that the cupping therapy is a must solution for such cases (Splenomegalies). Moreover, cupping can stimulate the reticuloendothelial cells to carry out its important immunity role against germs, parasites, fungi and protozoons. It is clear that cupping application according to its rules is a secondary spleen which forms a main assistant for the spleen in the blood filtration from all unwanted materials and spoiled and dead blood cells. So cupping Medicine is a very important protective of, and curing treatment in such cases of spleen problems.

The effect of Cupping on the liver:

When cupping removes the spoiled and senile corpuscles and the impurities from the blood, and it increases blood flow in all tissues and organs, consequently in the liver tissue. So, the liver cells will be activated and then the whole liver will be activated to perform its other functions in a complete performing. It will transform the cholesterol and the excessive triglycerides by its metabolic function, and stores the excessive sugar in blood with help from the pancreas in reducing glucose level to normal one in the diabetics. And the liver will be more active in rescuing the body from poisons, this activate all its systems including the brain and nervous system so the general health of body is better.

It also heightens the regeneration of spoiled tissues in the body because the liver is responsible for the production of the necessary protein for continuation of life and growth, it is clear that cupping medicine is a cure or main improving of all hepatic problems including all types of hepatitis, and prevents from or curing the hypertension of the portal vein and all resulting dangerous problems.

Prof. Dr. A. G. Jabakji, the specialist in neuromicroscopic surgery from Holland, says, "The implementation of cupping as it has been recommended is an explicit and clear entrance to complete health and good recovery. It supplies man with great power and energy by way of opening and cleaning the fine blood vessels within which blood precipitates and forms residues on its walls, and such a case is one of the causes of migraine, heart and liver diseases, and other ailments of the age." If we consider the hepatic Enzymes as a criterion for all treated cases where the levels of them are high, the findings are; after cupping they return to their normal levels.

Effect of the Cupping therapy on immunity:

The cupping therapy increases the ability and activity of the immunity system due to the increased activity of the reticals-endothelial system, and the good blood flow through the tissues and organs heightens the immunity of the body because that the pathogens in the body are more subjected to the immunity system unites. Interferon is the quickest defensive line to be formed and secreted after the exposure of the body to any virus. Prof. Kanteel says, "That the leukocytes can produce interferon in a rate exceeding ten times more than the other body cells produce." The tests of cupping blood showed a presence of very slight rate of leukocytes in it in addition to its great effect in producing the immunity defensive cells as the phagocytes which destroy pathogenic agents. This development in the stem (initial) blood cells go toward leukocytes formation, that the case of body demanding increasing in white blood cells in order to defend the body against the pathogenic agents. Here we can say: cupping keeps the leukocytes (there is just a very slight rate of leukocytes in cupping blood) and activates its production that helps in producing interferon in abundant quantities to face the hepatic virus or cancer cells.

The Effect of cupping on the heart and the blood thrombi:

In this era we hear every day about a sudden death and paralysis. These incidents are attributed to blood clots which are nothing but an agglomeration of red and white corpuscles, platelets and fibrin fibers crowded together at the ramifications of arteries to form a clot, its main happening is hypertension. The cupping operation has a great preventive role as it was mentioned in some of Hadiths that it prevents (hyperemia). In the dictionary of "Lissan Al-Arab" hyperemia means "agitation and increase," This description applies also on arterial hypertension and real increase in red corpuscles (poly Cythemia vera; Erythremia).

The disturbance of the cardiac system may be caused by ischemia or oxyachrestia. Also myocardia infarction is due to ischemia resulting from arterial stenosis (arteriosclerosis) and the thrombi themselves when they are in these coronary arteries.

The angina pectoris is generated when there is a decrease in supplying the heart tissue with the necessary Oxygen. Because the fat precipitations have partly blocked up the coronary artery. Then the high level of arterial hypertension may lead to complications such as: cardiac insufficiency, angina pectoris and encephala vascular incident. The long arterial hypertension may cause heart enlargement, and atherosclerosis. So, applying cupping is the best solution to prevent and treat such cases, as cupping decreases the level of fat (triglyceride, cholesterol) in blood to normal one, gets rid of hypertension and increases the blood flow through heart tissue after cleaning the arteries and preventing them from atherosclerosis.

The Effect of Cupping on the Digestive system:

The blood stagnation in the veins of the stomach and the intestines destroys their secretive and absorption functions and that will lead to severe bleeding, especially the vessels of the stomach, the intestines, the esophagus and the rectum, and blood clots in the legs and feet, hemorrhoids, and severe menstruation "in women", all of what mentioned above leads blood pressure to go down. So, cupping therapy activates the blood flow and consequently prevents blood from the in the digestive system. Therefore we cupping prevents and treats all the above mentioned cases. Most patients have their problems with hemorrhoids come to an end after performing cupping. The heightening blood pressure with a sluggish blood circulation leads to harm the biliary tracts and increases the density of the bile. Here cholesterol and bilirubin start to crystallize and that hinders the circulation of the arterial blood.

Whereas the compactness of the aged red corpuscles and their precipitation result in the impeded circulation in portal vein. Eventually, the tension of the portal vein heightens to push a part of the blood to the peripheral circulation round the liver through vessels anastomosis, consequently the spleen congests and enlarges and also does the venous vessels in the pancreas leading to its atrophy and its inability to do its functions. This is what we have seen. In fact, the cupping operation is a prevention and cure for all these problems and saves us from the trouble.

The Effect of Cupping Operation on the Nervous System, especially, the Brain:

The vascular incidents of the brain can be referred to two things:

- The ischemia and its rate (80%).
- Bleeding and its rate (20%).

If the ischemia extends, it will lead to brain congestion and results in hemiplegia. And this what we have avoided its occurrence by performing a therapy.

The cupping therapy is helpful in regulating the blood coming to the brain. It is also found to be useful in cases of memory weakness and lack of concentration. It also helps in controlling and regulating feelings and affections. Cupping was also mentioned for its usefulness for epilepsy and in improving the hearing if the cause was ischemia, and the stability resulting from lack of the coming blood.

The Effect of Cupping Operation on Diabetes:

One of the factors of heightening the rate of sugar in blood is ischemic the case where the body is stimulated to liberate glucose in order to raise the activity of its organs. Unluckily, the cause is not in the burning or in the ability, but the ischemic meager. And this explains the secret of immediate recovery for diabetic people soon after performing the operation. The activity of the liver and pancreas share much in reducing the level of sugar in the blood. This is what we have seen while performing the therapy.

The Effect of Cupping therapy on the Eye Diseases:

Cupping, while playing its role in removing from the blood all that impedes its movement and prevents it from stagnation. In this way, it activates the blood circulation and improves the perfusion of tissues and organs, and at the same time, it raises the activities of the various organs and systems of the body in addition to what result from the rearrangement of the hormone secretion leading to raise the immunity and defense of the body and its systems, especially the brain, the optic nerve, and the retina improving, in his way, the general state of the eyesight.

The Effect of Cupping therapy on the Kidneys:

The two kidneys usually do their duty of cleaning the body from nitrogen products, regulate the concentration of sodium, and metabolize the body liquids. They also concentrate the ions in blood and the balance of PH in the body, the deficiency of blood perfusion to the kidneys breaks down the kidneys from doing their elimination function and that may cause kidney failure, or to fall victim of Boliva disease which affects the brain and kills its cells. Cupping eliminates the ischemia from the kidneys and encourages them to function their duties to the best and that will increase the resistance of the body against diseases in general.

Effect of the Cupping Operation on the Malignant Disease of the Time (Cancer):

The accumulation of blood impurities will affect negatively the flow of blood, the perfusion of the tissues and organs will decrease, then the heart will exert more effort to secure their requirements. When the outpouring of blood lessens from the liver, the blood impurities deviates it from its most important duty in removing poisonous materials.

The function of the spleen will be lowered in its immunity level in producing antibodies and in straining the blood from strange elements. The work of the systems will recede little by little. The person will not immediately feel these changes in his body until old age when situations worsen, the troubles appear, and diseases creep upon him. For this reason we find that the rate of infection in cancer is greater in aged people than it is in others. All this is due to the absence of cupping. When the outside factors, such as chemical and radiological elements, and psychological impacts, the body becomes a prey for these aggressors. This is not all, for the body cells proliferated madly until they revolted against this body, and it was cancer. Any disturbance in the systems of the body leads to disturbance in the hormone disequilibrium with the outside factors. But the result was bigger than a weak immunity system weakened by ischemia. The organism recognizes the cancerous cells and considers them strange and forms antibodies against them seeking to control this tumor and trying to stop its diffusion, and the tumor appears when the equilibrium tends to the advantage of the cancerous cells.

Cancer has grown up when its cells overcome the immunity system, and the immunity system is linked with the systems and organs of the body, and the whole forms an integrated unity. If the liver worked in a high competence and saved the body from poisons, and stored, analyzed and combined, and the spleen accomplished its turn by changing its immunity cells, the T-B phagocytes, into secreting cells for globulins, and the humeral immunity was strengthened, and the two kidneys were purifying and organizing the mineral salts in a high efficiency as the rest systems and organs of the body do, then the body will restrain all outside effects and remains safe and sound. Statistics have shown that persons, who took medicines to inhibit immunity when they performed renal transplantation operations, were more exposed to infection by cancerous tumors than normal ones in a rate that reaches (35) times more. Some cases were found in the Americans that (74%) of those people infected by cancer were complaining from viral hepatitis. The owner of a weak liver is more exposed to primary hepatic cancer. One of the studies showed that the rate of infection by hepatic cancer between males was higher than it was with females by (6) times. And this is the result of menstruation, that "Divine Cupping".

Studies have shown that the tumor cells in the blood circulation, which saved them-selves from damage, become a malignant dissemination whose rate did not exceed one cell out of ten thousand cells from the total tumor cells because the effect of immunity was strong in the blood medium. For this reason doctors started using anticoagulins to stop spreading of the cancerous cells. Cupping heightens the efficiency of the immunity system in general and save us the trouble, and of the spoiled corpuscles and of the blood impurities. It reduces the blood viscosity, and raises its liquidity in a normal way without artificial induction, and the induction of bone marrows to produce more immunity cells.

This is what the lab studies have proved and were affirmed by our lab team. The spleen concentrates itself to practice its immunity role, and the systems of the body are rehabilitated, and heightened their capacities by cupping therapy and in bettering the patient's situation or a certain recovery of this malignant disease. The cupping therapy improves the eyesight resulting from insufficiency of perfusion and lessen clotting of blood by removing the extra congestive blood and eventually it lessens brain clots, and in reducing arterial pressure, it lessens occurrence of brain hemorrhage, and in strengthening immunity, it also lessens occurrence of neuro-immunity lesions. In no doubt, science will discover other advantages for cupping in advance of time to show that it is an excellent helpful device in treating a number of diseases.

Physiological effects:

Cupping assists the actions of Physis. Practitioners of cupping contend that this process strengthens the immune system, so encouraging the optimum functioning of the body. Cupping assists the liver by increasing blood perfusion, so removing the metabolic load imposed by the disease and perhaps any drugs used to treat the disease. It also supports the immune system, by acting on the reticulo-endothelial system to help it in opposing the actions of invading microbes. In addition, cupping supports the nervous system, by helping to reverse ischaemia, which can lead to conditions characterized by cerebro-metabolic insufficiency, such as memory disturbances, epilepsy and emotional conditions. Finally, cupping supports the renal system, by helping to reverse the ischaemia which underlies many disorders. Cupping is also involved in the release of cortisol and serotonin, important mediators in pain and stress. Cupping also stimulates acupuncture points, and releases biological opioids called endorphins.

Clinical value

The benefits of cupping have been extensively researched and documented. Cupping is recommended for people with recurring, refractory headaches, skin disorders, stomach pain, boils, disorders of the heart and circulation, such as varicose veins and hypertension, joint and neck pains, for example, arthritis and rheumatism, diarrhoea and vomiting, menstrual cramps, bronchitis, colds, asthma, infertility, impotence, and haemorrhoids, amongst other ailments. The clinical benefits of cupping continue for several days after the procedure.

Chapter 9

INDICATIONS OF CUPPING POINTS/PLACES FOR VARIOUS DISEASES

INDICATIONS OF CUPPING POINTS/PLACES FOR VARIOUS DISEASES

Sites and procedures of Cupping

S.No.	Points of Application	Uses
1.	Nape of the neck	Heaviness of eyelids, Itch of eyes.
2.	Shoulders	Pain in the upper arms and Throat
3.	The leg (Hijamate saaq)	Cleanses blood, Provokes menstrual flow
4.	Over the joints	Inflammatory masses in the upper part of thigh
5.	Front of thigh	Orchitis, Leg ulcers
6.	In inner of thigh	Poadagra, Piles, Bladder, Renal congestion
7.	In popliteal space	Aneurysm, Septic ulcers of leg and foot

8.	Over malleoli (ankle bone)	Sciatica, Piles, Podagra and retained menses
9.	Over the outer side of hips	Inguinal hernia
10.	Under the chin	Cleanses of the teeth, facse, throat, head and jaws
11.	Over the ankle	Amenorrhoea, sciatica and gout

Some cupping instruments

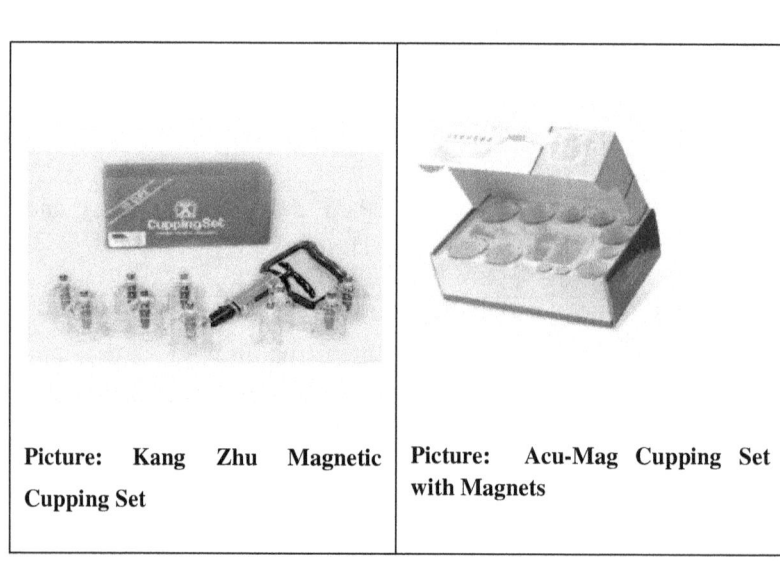

Picture: Kang Zhu Magnetic Cupping Set	**Picture: Acu-Mag Cupping Set with Magnets**

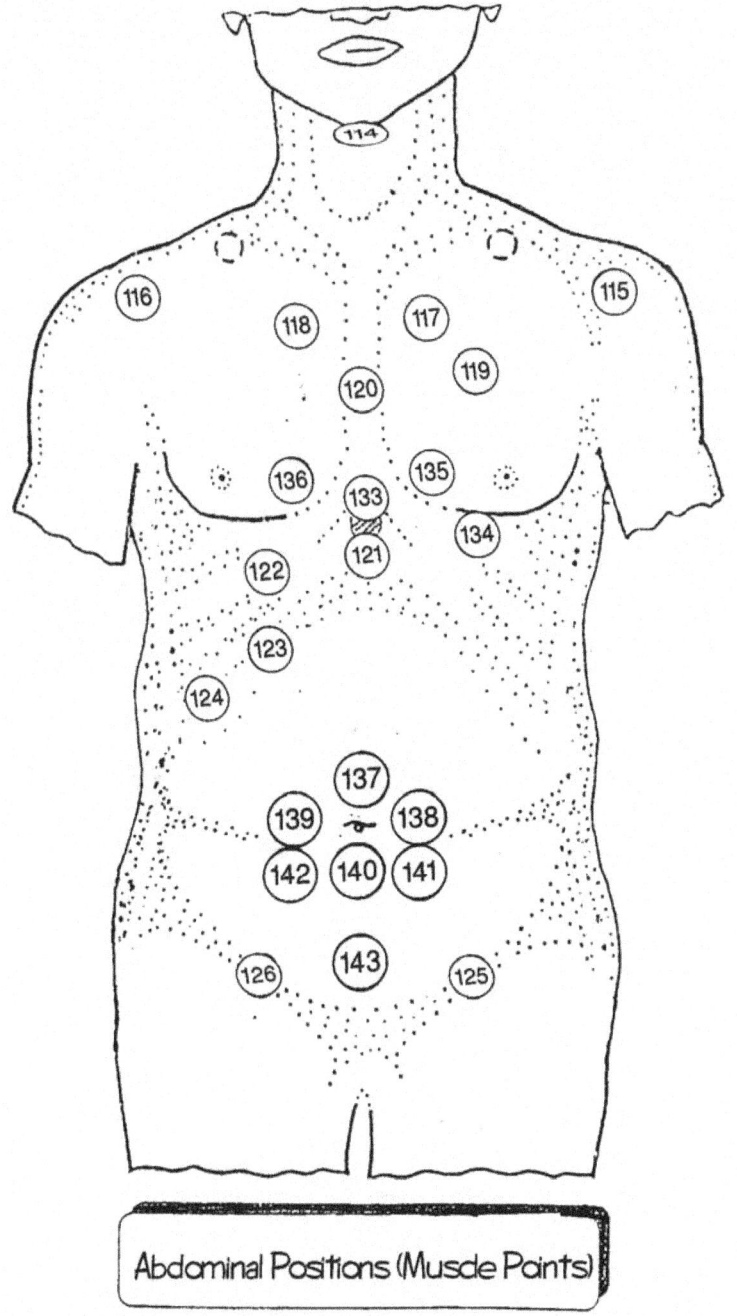

Abdominal Positions (Muscle Points)

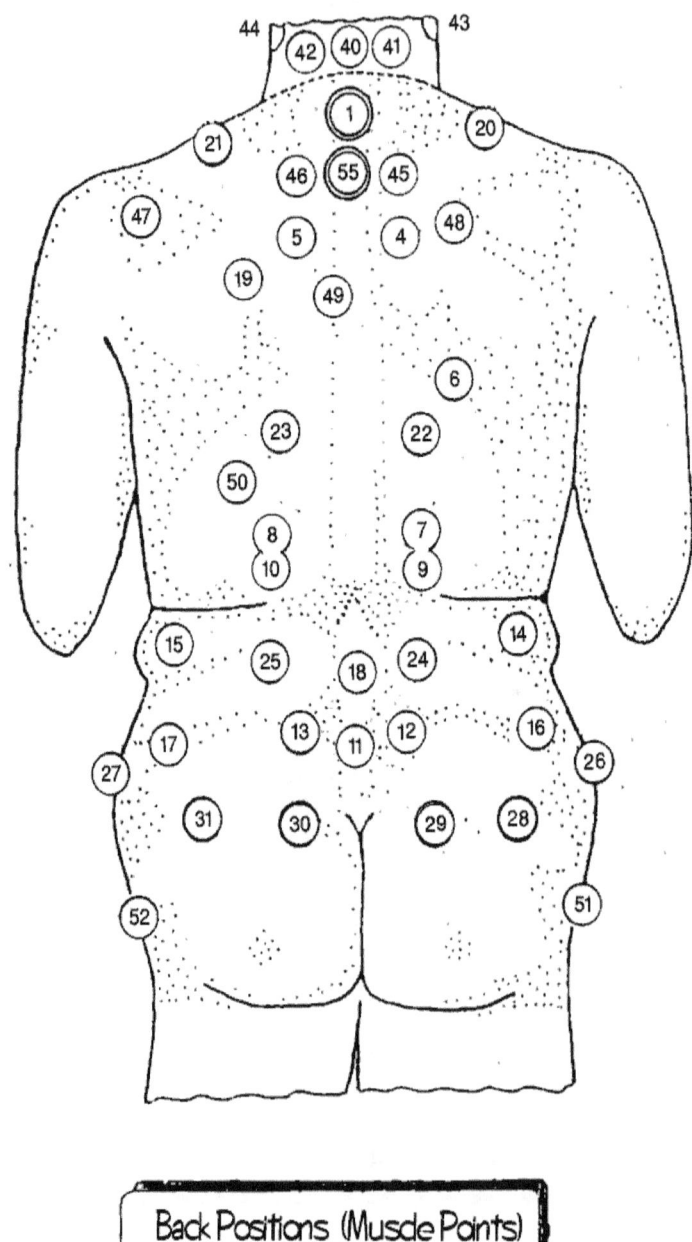

Back Positions (Muscle Points)

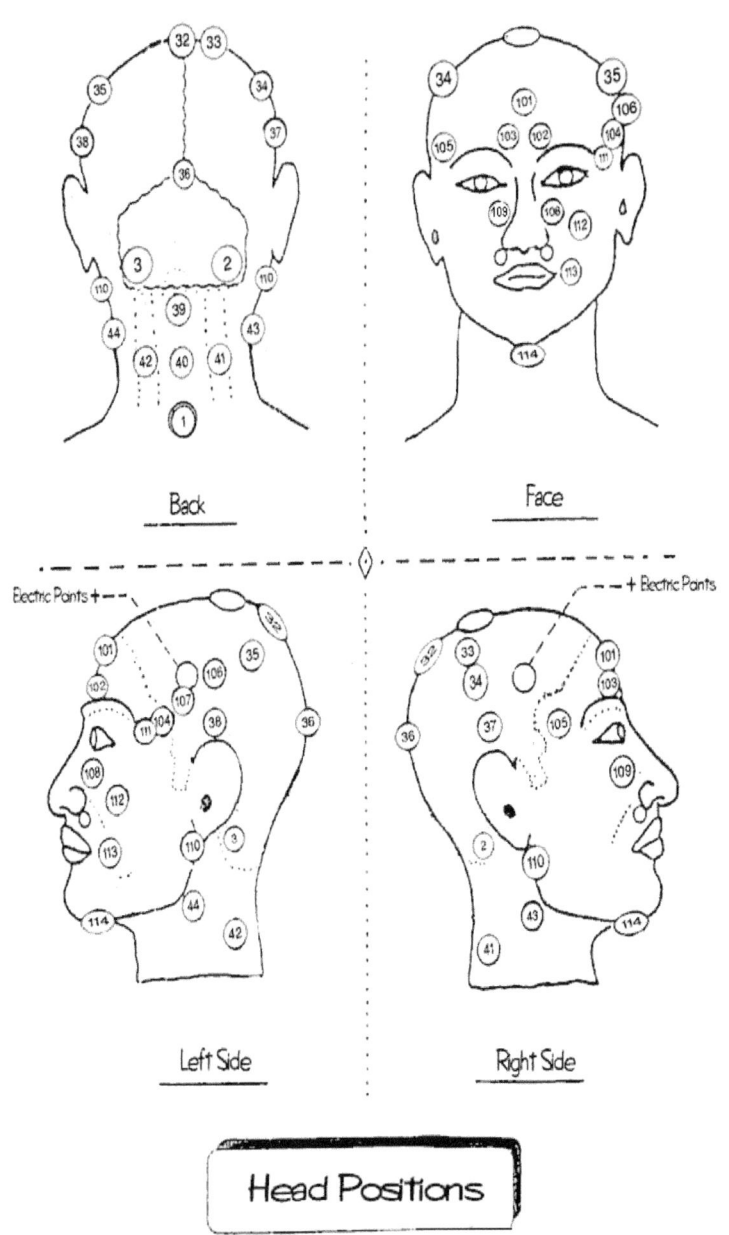

Back

Face

Left Side

Right Side

Head Positions

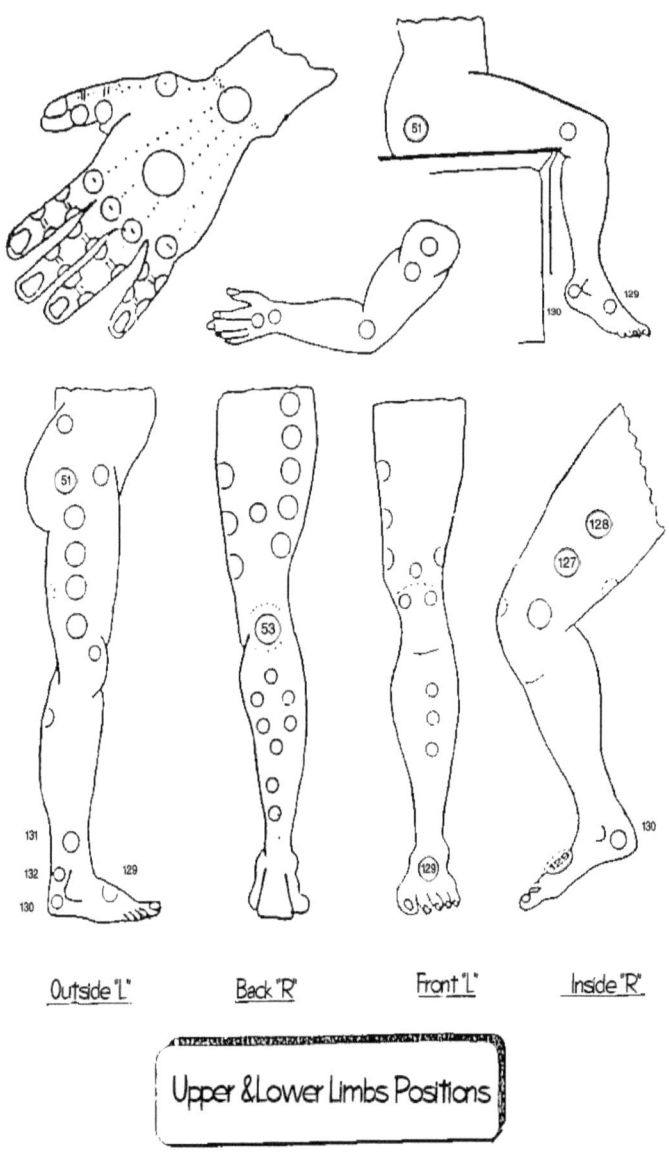

Outside "L"   Back "R"   Front "L"   Inside "R"

Upper & Lower Limbs Positions

Group (A)

- **Rheumatism (painful joints)** (points 1, 55, in addition to all areas of pain).
- **Roughness of knee** (points 1, 55, 11, 12, 13 and cupping around the knee and you may add 53, 54).
- **Oedema (swollen tissue due to build up of fluid)** (points 1, 55, 130, the right and left side of the heel and you may add 9, 10).
- **Sciatic pain (nerve pain from the buttock which goes down the leg)** (for the right leg) (points 1, 55, 11, 12, 26, 51 and places of pain on the leg especially the beginning and the end of the muscle) (for the left leg) (points 1, 55, 11, 13, 27, 52 and places of pain on the leg especially the beginning and the end of the muscle).
- **Back pain** (positions 1, 55 and cupping on both sides of the spine and places of pain).
- **Neck/shoulder pain** (points 1, 55, 40, 20, 21 and places of pain).

- **Gout (swollen joints due to excess uric acid)** (points 1, 55, 28, 29, 30, 31, 121 and places of pain).
- **Rheumatoid Arthritis** (points 1, 55, 120, 49, 36 and all large and small joints).
- **Paralysis of one half of the body (Hemiplegia)** (points 1, 55, 11, 12, 13, 34 or 35 and all the injured joints, massage daily).
- **Paralysis of all four limbs (Quadriplegia)** (points 1, 55, 11, 12, 13, 34, 35, 36 and all body joints and daily massage).
- **Immune system deficiency** (points 1, 55, 120, 49).
- **Muscle spasm** several dry cupping around the affected muscle.
- **Poor blood circulation** (points 1, 55, 11 and ten cups on both sides of the spine from the top to the bottom in addition to taking a teaspoon of pure organic, raw, apple cider vinegar and honey every other day).
- **Tingling arms** (points 1, 55, 40, 20, 21, arm muscles and affected joints).

- **Tingling feet** (points 1, 55, 11, 12, 13, 26, 27, feet joints and affected muscles).
- **Abdominal pain** (points 1, 55, 7, 8 and dry cupping on 137, 138, 139, 140, as well as dry cupping on the back opposite to the pain).

(Dry Cupping means without any incisions/scratches) .

Group (B)

Important Note: The following points are arranged according to their importance. Sometimes, the cupping therapist does not need to use all of the points and sometimes he/she has to use them all, depending on the condition of the disease.

- **Hemorrhoids (swollen vessels around anus)** (points 1, 55, 121, 11, 6 and dry cupping on 137, 138, 139).
- **Anal Fistula (opening in skin near anus, due to formation of a channel through which fluid leaks)** (points 1, 55, 6, 11, 12, 13 and cupping around the anus and above the fistula hole).
- **Prostate and Erectile dysfunction, ED (male impotence and urinary difficulty**

due to enlarged prostate gland)(points 1, 55, 6, 11, 12, 13) and you may add for ED 125, 126, 131 on both legs, and dry cupping on 140, 143).

- **Chronic coughs and lung diseases** (points 1, 55, 4, 5, 120, 49, 115, 116, 9, 10, 117, 118, 135, 136, and two cups below both knees).

- **Hypertension (high blood pressure)** (points 1, 55, 2, 3, 11, 12, 13, 101, 32, 6, 48, 9, 10, 7, 8, and you may replace 2, 3 with 43, 44).

- **Stomach problems and ulcers** (points 1, 55, 7, 8, 50, 41, 42 and dry cupping on 137, 138, 139, 140).

- **Renal (kidney) disease** (points 1, 55, 9, 10, 41, 42 and dry cupping on 137,140).

- **Irritable bowel syndrome (abdominal cramps and discomfort characterized by bloating and trapped wind and alternating bouts of diarrhea and constipation, often related to anxiety)** (points 1, 55, 6, 48, 7, 8, 14, 15, 16, 17, 18, 45, 46 and dry cupping on 137).

- **Chronic constipation (long term difficulty with opening bowels)** (points 1, 55, 11, 12, 13, 28, 29, 30, 31).
- **Diarrhea** (dry cupping on 137, 138, 139, 140).
- **Involuntary urination (bed wetting)** (after the age of five: dry cupping on 137, 138, 139, 140, 142, 143, 125, 126).
- **Depression, withdrawal, insomnia (inability to sleep), psychological conditions and nervousness** (points 1, 55, 6, 11, 32 and below the knees).
- **Angiospasm and Arteriosclerosis (narrowing of the blood vessels due to muscular spasm or fatty deposits)**(points 1, 55, 11) (cupping points are on the places of pain in addition to a teaspoon of pure, organic, raw, apple cider vinegar and honey every other day).
- **Inflammation in the lining of the stomach (gastritis)** (points 1, 55, 121).
- **Excessive sleep** (points 1, 55, 36) in addition to a teaspoon of pure, organic, raw, apple cider vinegar and honey every other day).

- **Food allergies** (one dry cup using a light suction directly on the umbilicus pit [belly button]).
- **Sores, leg and thigh abscesses (pus filled spots) and itching of iliac fossae (itching in hip area)** (points 1, 55, 129, 120).

Group (C)

Important Note: The following points are arranged according to their importance. Sometimes, the cupping therapist does not need to use all of the points and sometimes he/she has to use them all depending on the condition of the disease.

- **Heart disease** (points 1, 55, 19, 119, 7, 8, 46, 46, 47, 133, 134).
- **Diabetes** (points 1, 55, 6, 7, 8, 22, 23, 24, 25, 120, 49) note: the area of cupping should be applied with black seed oil or honey for 3 days.
- **Liver and gall bladder disease** (points 1, 55, 6, 48, 41, 42, 46, 51, 122, 123, 124 and 5 cups on the right, outer leg).
- **Varicose veins (enlarged, unsightly superficial veins) on the legs** (points 1,

55, 28, 29, 30, 31, 132 and around the veins but NOT over the veins).

- **Varicocele (enlarged unsightly veins on scrotum of male)** (points 1, 55, 6, 11, 12, 13, 28, 29, 30, 31, 125, 126).

- **Elephantiasis (swollen leg due to blockage of lymph channels)** note: the patient should rest for 2 days before cupping. He/She should also raise his/her affected leg up and then place it in warm water for two hours prior to cupping (points 1, 55, 11, 12, 13, 120, 49, 121 and around the affected leg from the top of the leg to the bottom in addition to 125, 126, 53, 54).

- **Skin diseases** (points 1, 55, 49, 120, 129, 6, 7, 8, 11 and cupping on the affected areas).

- **Overweight** (points 1, 55, 9, 10, 120, 49 and areas of desired weight loss), daily massage cupping over area of desired weight loss.

- **Underweight** (points 1, 55, 121).

- **Cellulite** daily massage cupping over affected area.
- **Infertility** (points 1, 55, 6, 11, 12, 13, 120, 49, 125, 126, 143, 41, 42).
- **Thyroid disease** (points 1, 55, 41, 42).

Group (D)

- **Headaches** (points 1, 55, 2, 3) and you may replace points 2, 3 with 43, 44. If it is caused by **eye strain** add 104, 105 and 36. If it is caused by **nasal sinuses** add 102, 103 and 114. If it is caused by **high blood pressure** add 11, 101 and 32. If it is caused by **constipation** add 28, 29, 30 and 31. If it is caused by **a cold** add 120, 4 and 5. If it is caused by a**stomach ache** add 7, 8. If it is caused by **the kidneys** add 9, 10. If it is caused by **menstruation** for women add 11, 12 and 13. If it is caused by **gall bladder** and **liver** add 6, 48. If it is caused by the **spine column** perform cupping on the spine. If it is caused by tension add 6, 11 and 32. If it is caused by **anemia** add 120, 49 and take one teaspoon of black honey (molasses) with a quarter of a teaspoon of ground fenugreek and 7 ground black seeds daily. If the headache is due to **tumors** in the brain, cupping should be performed on the area of pain on the head).

- **Migraine (severe headache associated with nausea and visual disturbance)** (points 1, 55, 2, 3, 106 and area of pain).

- **Diseases of the eyes (retina, eye disorder, blurred vision, atrophy of the eye nerves, glaucoma (Blue Water), cataract (White Water) and weak eye, eye inflammation and secretion of tears and eye sensitivity** (points 1, 55, 36, 101, 104 , 105, 9, 10, 34, 35, above the eyebrows and on the hair line above the forehead).

- **Tonsils, throat, gums, teeth, and the middle ear problems (dizziness, nausea and ringing in ears)** (points 1, 55, 20, 21, 41, 42, 120, 49, 114, 43, 44).

- **Weakness of hearing and inflammation of hearing nerve, tinnitus (ringing sensation** in ears) (points 1, 55, 20, 21, 37, 38 and behind the ear).

- **Nasal sinuses** (points 1, 55, 102, 103, 108, 109, 36, 14 and on the hair line).
- **Neuritis (inflammation) of the fifth and seventh nerves** (points 1, 55, 110, 111, 112, 113, 114 and on the affected area).
- **To stimulate the system of perception (encourage awareness)** (points 1, 55, 2, 3, 32).
- **Clinical Memory Loss** (important: if point 39 is cupped unnecessarily it may cause damage to the memory. Also its unnecessary repetition may increase memory loss (point 39 occipital prominence).
- **Mute (unable to speak)** (points 1, 55, 36, 33, 107, 114).
- **To help stop smoking** (points 1, 55, 106, 11, 32).
- **Convulsion (fits)** (points 1, 55, 101, 36, 32, 107 on both sides, 114, 11, 12, 13).
- **For the treatment of mental retardation** (points 1, 55, (101 only once) 36, 32, 2, 3, 120, 49, 11, 12, 13).

- **Atrophy (loss) of brain cells (oxygen deficiency)** (points 1, 55, 101, 36, 32, 34, 35, 11 and perform cupping on the joints, muscles and neck, 43 and 44 on the front and back. Eat honey and royal jelly. Perform massage cupping daily).

Group (E) Gynecological

Important warning: pregnant women should avoid cupping during pregnancy except if they are over-due and wish to go into labour. In this case, they should have dry and massage cupping between the knee and ankle on both legs. Cupping a pregnant woman may cause miscarriage.

- **Hemorrhage (vaginal bleeding)** (points 1, 55, (3 dry cups under each breast daily until bleeding ceases).
- **Amenorrhea (absence of periods)** (points 1, 55, 129, (131 from the outside), 135, 136) .
- **Brownish Secretion** 3 dry cups under each breast daily until secretion ceases (points 1, 55, 120, 49, 11, 12, 13 and 143). If secretion has no smell, no colour

or itching, perform cupping on (points 1, 55, 9, 10, 41, 42, 11, 12, 13, 143).

- **Menstruation (period) problems** (points 1, 55 (dry cupping on 125, 126, 137, 138, 139, 140, 141, 142, 143).

- **To stimulate the ovaries** (points 1, 55, 11, (dry cupping on 125, 126).

- **Pain after a uterus (womb) operation, menstrual (period) pain, the problems of ligation of the fallopian tube (tube being tied/blocked), milk existence in the breast without being pregnant and menopausal symptoms (depression, nervousness, psychological conditions, acute uterus)** (points 1, 55, 6, 48, 11, 12, 13, 120, 49) (Dry Cupping on 125, 126). To regulate the menses, it is preferred to perform cupping on the second day of the menses.

Cupping places on the back

1, the shoulder, the seventh vertebra (bone of spine) of the neck.

2 & 3, the area between the ears, the back of the head where hair grows or on the sides of the neck.

4 & 5, the air door between the two ribs upwards in the branching of the tracheae (main windpipe) and the bronchus (smaller windpipe).

6, the gall bladder at the peripheral of the right rib toward the spine.

7 & 8, on the stomach place at the middle of the back opposite to the stomach on the spinal sides.

9 & 10, the kidney centre under **7 & 8** on the middle of the back.

11, lumbar vertebrae - a prominent bone at the lower back of the vertebra column.

12 & 13, on the sides of **11,** slightly upward, 5cm away from the spine.

14, 15, 16 & 17, the colon, almost on the colon corners from the back and **18** of the middle of the spine.

19, the heart, opposite to the heart from the back and almost on the left rib side.

20 & 21, tonsils triangle that lies in the area between the neck and the shoulder with a slight bending to the back.

22 & 23, above the pancreas gland under the rib end.

24 & 25, at the beginning of the lower half of the back.

26 & 27, bilaterally at the sides of the iliac bone.

28, 29, 30 & 31, at the upper part of the buttocks.

32, on the middle of the head.

33, on the right part of the hair near the forehead or the hair line.

34 & 35, the right and left part of the brain (at the temporal sides of the brain) as well as the occipital bone.

36, the cerebellum (occipital) prominent bone on the head.

37 & 38, nearly 3cm above the ears.

39, prominent occipital bone, the deep area at the back of the head where cupping is prohibited, except in necessary cases.

40, in the middle of the back of the neck.

41 & 42, on the back of the head to the right and the left.

43 & 44, the sides of the neck.

45 & 46, nearly 3cm above the air trachea **(4-5)**.

47, on the left shoulder in addition to the heart.

48, on the right rib from upward, complementary to the gall bladder knot.

49, the immunity area from the back, between the two scapulae (shoulder blades).

50, 6cm slightly above **8,** for stomach ulcers.

51 & 52, the two thigh bones (femur), from both sides.

53 & 54, the inner part of the knee from the back.

55, almost 3cm under the shoulder.

Cupping places on the face and abdomen

101, the forehead on the place of worship in praying and it is better not to repeat it.

102 & 103, above the eyebrows from the inner part of the nasal sinuses.

104 & 105, on both sides of the brows and slightly upward for headaches and sight.

106, almost 6cm above the left ear to help give up smoking.

107, nearly 4cm above the cheeks to assist in speech.

108 & 109, on the sides of the nose for nasal sinuses.

110, under the ear from the right and left.

111, 112 & 113, near the eye and the cheek and near the lip to treat the fifth and sixth nerve.

114, under the chin and it has many benefits.

115 & 116, under the ends of the clavicle (collar bone) from the outside and on the shoulders.

117 & 118, under the clavicle (collar bone) from the inside, on the chest.

119, the heart, under the middle of the left clavicle (collar bone) using four fingers of the patient himself.

120, sternum bone (breastplate), in the middle of the chest.

121, first part of the stomach directly under the chest bone.

122, 123 & 124, above the liver, right of the belly.

125 & 126, between the belly and the thigh near the pubic hair area for involuntary urination, infertility...etc.

127 & 128, on the inner part of the thighs.

129, on the back of the feet to the right.

130, on the sides of the heel from inside and outside for edema.

131, above the heel bone nearly 5cm from the outside.

132, varicocele.

133, almost 2cm above the stomach mouth and near the end of the chest bone.

134, under the left breast.

135 & 136, 5cm away from the breast nipple from the inside for the lungs.

137, 138, 139 & 140, above, right, left and under the umbilicus (belly button).

141, & 142, Right and left of **140**.

143, above the bladder.

Chapter 10

CLINICAL RESEARCHES DONE ON CUPPING THERAPY

CLINICAL RESEARCHES DONE ON CUPPING THERAPY

Numerous RCTs on cupping therapy have been conducted and published during the past decades. This review showed that cupping has potential effect in the treatment of herpes zoster and other specific conditions. However, further rigorously designed trials on its use for other conditions are warranted.

In 2001 "prepared under the supervision of Dr. M. Nabeel Al-Shareef, the prior dean of the faculty of Pharmacy" The study was preformed according to the scientific rules which the great Humane Scholar Mohammad Amin Sheikho deduced from the noble prophetic traditions. These rules state that cupping should be applied: In the early morning, on fasting, in the springtime, during the second half of the lunar months corresponding to April and May (in the

Mediterranean countries as Syria), for men over twenty years old, and for women over menopause.

The research included 300 cases which have been studied by a laboratory medical team and a clinical medical team. The findings of the study were as follows:

1- In cases of hypertension, the blood pressure decreased to its normal limit.

2- In cases of hypotension, the blood pressure increased to its normal limit.

3- The electrocardiograms showed a great improvement, and graphically there was a return to normal situation in the segments slide.

4- Decrease to normal limits in ESR.

5- Moderation in the red corpuscles count.

6- In all cases of polycythemia (Erythremia), the value of hemoglobin decreased to its normal limit.

7- In all cases of low hemoglobin, its value increased to the normal limit. This denotes an activity in the body and a growth in its ability in producing benign young red corpuscles which help in more active and effective transporting of oxygen.

8- In 60% of the cases (cupped persons), there was a rise in leukocytes count within normal limits.

9- The count of leukocytes increased in 71,4% of cases of rheumatic diseases. This explains the instant recovery of the rheumatic patients and those who suffer from chronic inflammations after they use cupping.

10- Neutrophils count increased within normal limits in 100% of cases of rheumatic diseases.

11- In 83,3% of cases of asthma, the neutrophils count increased within normal limits.

12- Neutrophils count fall to normal limits in all cases of abnormal neutrophilia.

13- In cases of heart diseases, the neutrophils count fell to normal limits in the rate of 76,9% of the cases.

14- Rise in thrombocytes count in 50,6% of the cases.

15- In all cases of thrombocytopenia, the count of thrombocytes became normal.

16- In 50% of cases of essential thrombocytosis, the count decreased to normal limits.

17- Glucose level in blood decreased in 83,75 % of the cases, while it remained within its normal limits in the rest.

18- 92,5 % of cases of diabetic patients showed a decrease in glucose value.

19- Creatinine value in blood decreased in 66,66 % of the cases.

20- The quantity of creatinine contained in the cupping blood was high in all cases.

21- 78,57% of patients having a high level of creatinine in blood showed decrease in it.

22- The value of uric acid in blood fell in 66,66 % of the cases.

23- The level of uric acid in blood decreased, at the patients suffering from its rise, in 73,68 % of the cases.

24- The value of urea in blood decreased in 50,7 % of the cases.

25- Urea level in blood decreased in 80% of cases having a rise in it.

26- 80% of cases of high level of the liver Enzyme (SGPT) showed falling in it. This indicates that the liver has been activated after performing cupping

27- SGOT (a liver Enzyme) became lower in 80% of cases of patients having a high level of it. This explains the improvement that the electrocardiogram showed.

28- Alkaline phosphatase (a liver enzyme) decreased in 62,85 % of the cases where it was high.

29- The amylase level in blood became lower in 54,9 % of the cases.

30- In all cases of a high value of albumin in blood, the value returned to its normal limit.

31- The cholesterol level in blood became lower in 81,9 % of the cases.

32- Regarding the patients who had a high value of cholesterol in blood, the value decreased in 83,6 % of the cases.

33- The triglycerides level decreased in 75 % of the cases where it was high.

34- (K) and (Na) ions became normal in 90 % of the cases.

35- (Ca) ions became normal in 90 % of the cases.

36- /CPK/ decreased in 66,66 % of the cases where it was high.

37- The red blood cells in the cupping blood withdrawn from the upper part of the back were all of abnormal shapes: Hypochromasia - Burr - Target - Crenated - Spherocytes - Poikilocytes - Anisocytosis - Shistocytes - Teardrop cells - Acanthocytes.

38- The leukocytes count in the cupping blood did not come to one tenth of their count in the venous blood. This indicates that the cupping operation keeps the components of immunity system in the body.

39- In 66% of the cases, there was an increase in the iron level within its normal limits.

40- (T.I.B.C.) was very high in the cupping blood where it varied between (422) and (1057) while in the venous blood it ranges between (250) to (400). This indicates that there is a mechanism which prevents iron from getting out of the cupping scratches retaining it inside the body so as to take part in building new blood cells. This is possibly associated with an activity in the process of iron absorption in the intestines.

41- (CPK) became normal in 92,4 % of the cases.

42- (LDH) became normal in 93,75 % of the cases.

These extremely dazzling findings reflected too many cases of marvelous recovery which came as a proof of the grandeur of the prophetic science and the weighty wonderwork brought by the First Teacher our master Mohammad (cpth) and transported to us by the great Humane Scholar Mohammad Amin Sheikho.

43. 135 RCTs published from 1992 through 2010 were identified. The studies were generally of low methodological quality. Diseases for which cupping therapy was commonly applied were herpes zoster, facial paralysis (Bell palsy), cough and dyspnea, acne, lumbar disc herniation, and cervical spondylosis. Wet cupping was used in most trials, followed by retained cupping, moving cupping, and flash cupping. Meta-analysis showed cupping therapy combined with other TCM treatments was significantly superior to other treatments alone in increasing the number of cured patients with herpes zoster, facial paralysis, acne, and cervical spondylosis. No serious adverse effects were reported in the trials.

44. In March 2011 three systematic reviews were analyzed for the effectiveness of wet and dry cupping in which two out of three showed some evidence for effectiveness of cupping for pain. Favorable effects were shown when wet cupping was combined with adjuvant conventional treatments. However, one of the three reviews showed little effectivess for cupping for stroke rehabilitation. Few randomized control trials have been done to examine the effectiveness of cupping and many studies published are of low quality or have many limitations.

45. A study conducted by Ahmed and colleagues in order to evaluate the efficiency of cupping [hijama] therapy in management of rheumatoid arthritis. To sum up they concluded cupping [hijama] combined with conventional medical therapy has several advantages. It significantly reduces the laboratory markers of disease activity and it modulates the immune cellular conditions particularly of innate immune response NK cell % and adaptive cellular immune response SIL-20 (**Ahmed, Madbouly, Maklad Abu-Shady, 2005)**

46. Using a pre-post research design, 70 patients with chronic tension or migraine headache were treated with wet-cupping. Three primary outcome measures were considered at the baseline and 3 months following treatment: headache severity, days of headache per month, and use of medication. Results suggest that, compared to the baseline, mean headache severity decreased by 66% following wet-cupping treatment. Treated patients also experienced the equivalent of 12.6 fewer days of headache per month. We conclude that wet-cupping leads to clinical relevant benefits for primary care patients with headache. Possible mechanisms of wet-cupping's efficacy, as well as directions for future research are discussed.

47. Australian and Chinese researchers reviewed 135 studies on cupping therapy published between 1992 and 2010. They concluded that cupping therapy may be effective when combined with other treatments like acupuncture or medications in treating various diseases and conditions, such as: Herpes zoster, Acne, Facial paralysis, and cervical spondylosis.

Research had shown the clinical effectiveness of CT for both physical and psychological conditions. To date research has involved the use of small scale studies however recent publications from China, Middle East and Iran in the form of Randomized Control Trials and Systematic reviews have provided a solid foundation for further studies.

Chapter 11

SAFETY, PRELIMINARIES, PROCESS, PRECAUTION, AND CONTRAINDICATIONS OF CUPPING

SAFETY ASPECTS OF CUPPING

❖ The practitioner must wear disposable latex gloves whilst carrying out both types of cupping.

❖ Before cupping actually begins, the patient's blood pressure and pulse should be checked.

❖ The blades used for wet cupping incisions should be disposable.

❖ The incisions in wet cupping should be superficial, involving the epidermis only.

❖ The patient should be questioned on how he or she feels - any unusual sensation or fever.

❖ All other necessary safety measures should be in place.

The Cupping technique Preliminaries:

❖ In obese persons and in those suffering from thickened blood (polycytaemia), a hot bath 1 to 2 hours before cupping is recommended. This helps to stimulate blood flow to the skin, so makes cupping that much more effective.

❖ As cupping is performed on the naked skin, the treatment room should be comfortably warm

❖ Make sure the patient is relaxed and not suffering from any degree of anxiety

❖ Explain to the patient what you about to do, demonstrate if necessary on your own arm

❖ In order to achieve better contact between the cup and the skin, liberally apply a suitable massage oil to the cupping intended area

❖ The selected areas of skin may be shaved, so that a good seal between the cup and skin can be achieved.

❖ Patients about to undergo cupping (especially the wet version) should be advised to take a nutritional drink before the cupping.

❖ Pressure applied to cups will vary according to patients. For medium to large frame patients, and in patients where the cupping sites are endowed with excess fatty tissue, the pressure can be increased. This ensures that the area beneath the glass will respond at a faster rate than on patients who are leaner, and with less fatty tissue.

❖ Cupping can also be carried out in parallel to massage. Choose the best position suitable for the patient and you as sudden movements are not recommended.

❖ The location to be treated is important in deciding the position of the patient. If the cupping is to be performed on the back, the most comfortable position will be prone on a bed or flat surface area; if on the stomach, a supine position is preferred. For the face, knees, neck and shoulders, a sitting position in a chair may be chosen. For the elderly, severe asthmatics or patients who have recently suffered form any heart conditions, an upright sitting position should always be preferred.

The process:

❖ The vacuum in the glass or hard plastic suction cup is usually created in one of two different ways.

❖ In the traditional method, the cup is heated by a flame from an alcohol soaked cotton pad or taper, then applied immediately to the skin. As the oxygen burns up, a vacuum is created "sealing" the jar to the skin. The device can be released easily by hand. These days, a hand operated vacuum pump is attached to the glass cup, and suction applied by manual action.

❖ The appropriate sized cups should be used.

❖ Generally, the cups should be placed on flat sections of the skin (which is usually hair-free, with no bony protuberances, and relatively thick).

❖ When more than one cup is used simultaneously, the cups should be separated by 1-2 centimeters.

❖ If wet cupping is to be carried out, the site selected for cup application will be incised superficially with a small blade (lancet). A stinging, but not usually painful, sensation will be experienced.

❖ The cup is then applied, and the air within will be evacuated with a small hand-held pump. This will draw 20 to 100mls blood into the cup, depending on the skin thickness of the application zone. After this, bleeding stops automatically, as haemostatic mechanisms come into operation.

❖ The process lasts for around 15 to 20 minutes from application of the cup.

❖ During cupping, the patient must remain as still as possible.

❖ Precautions need to be taken on when and where the cups are placed, and for how long they are applied.

Afterwards:

❖ An antiseptic cream should be applied to the incisions after cupping is terminated. The use of honey is not only effective as an antiseptic but also assists in the healing of the skin.

❖ Adequate nutritious liquids should be taken after cupping.

❖ Solid food intake should be avoided, if possible, for at least 3 hours.

❖ No shower or bathing should be carried out for 12 hours after cupping.

❖ Sexual activity should be refrained from for at least one day.

❖ After cupping, the following signs may be evident: Redness of the skin (erythema) which disappears after a few weeks, Slight itching, as the healing process takes place, at the cupping sites may develop and persist for a few days. Scratching should be discouraged. Light scarring as part of the healing process.

Contra-indications and Precautions to cupping therapy

Cupping Therapy has no major side effects aside from minimal discomfort due to the method of application of skin cuts to the patient. In cases where the patient's pain threshold is low, a local anaesthetic is usually administered. Also other possible minor side effects that may occur is the feeling of slight light headedness post Cupping Therapy, this is similar to the sensation one feels after having had blood taken from the doctor, as Cupping Therapy encourages blood flow to the cupped region (hyperaemia), one may therefore feel warmer and hotter as a result of vasodilatation (widening of blood vessel) taking place and slight sweating may occur. Again this can be attributed to sound scientific rationale and there is no cause for concern.

Pregnant women or menstruating women, cancer (metastatic) patients and patients with bone fractures or muscle spasms are also believed to be contra-indicated. Also, Cupping Therapy cannot be applied to a site of DVT (Deep Vein Thrombosis), where there are ulcers, arteries or places where a pulse can be felt (Chirali, 1999,).

Contrary to some claims, Cupping therapy cannot cure all diseases, and the mere fact that the Prophet (saw) utilised this treatment doesn't promote its value to a universal cure. Indeed the Prophet (peace and blessings be upon him) informed there was 'cure in it' and we should thus attempt to attain maximum benefit from it, and he never said to 'cure all illnesses from it'. Therefore it is the responsibility of the practitioner to be medically educated and well versed with the practice of al-Hijamah and the indications/contra-indications a treatment like Hijamah has. Although the practice of al-Hijamah should be advocated and the practice of the great Sunnah re-established, caution needs to be exercised against false attributions to the potential of Cupping Therapy. The Blessed Prophet warned us "He who introduces something new to Islam, which is not of it, will have it rejected'.

Although there are no firm contraindications to cupping, it should be used with circumspection in children, seriously ill patients, those with abnormally low blood pressure, and the aged. In these cases cupping can be done with discretion, and under special and defined circumstances.

- ❖ Dry cupping is not recommended for children below the age of 3 years.
- ❖ Wet cupping should be avoided in children below the age of 6 years.
- ❖ Wet cupping should not be carried out in patients above 65 years of age, although dry cupping can be used in the elderly.
- ❖ Precautions should be observed for menstruating women.
- ❖ It is not advisable to apply cupping to the patient with skin ulcers, oedema, or on an areas overlying large blood vessels or even varicose veins
- ❖ In addition, patients with high fever or who suffer from convulsions should not be cupped.

❖ Cupping should not be applied to the abdominal and sacral regions of the pregnant women.

❖ Wet cupping should never be applied to the female breast, unless absolutely necessary.

❖ Cupping on the neck or on the occipital bone is not advised. This can cause problems with eyesight and memory.

❖ Cupping on the forehead is likewise not advocated, as this can lead to emotional instability.

❖ Care should be taken with wet cupping of anaemic patients, or those susceptible to spontaneous bleeding.

❖ Cupping should not be done on patients who are visibly fatigued (physically or mentally), very hungry/thirsty, distraught, or who have overindulged in alcohol.

Chapter 12

FREQUENTLY ASKED QUESTIONS

FREQUENTLY ASKED QUESTIONS

a) Is cupping a cure for every disease?

Cupping is a cure for every disease if performed in its correct time. The Messenger (p.b.u.h) said, "Indeed in cupping there is a cure." [**Saheeh Muslim (5706)**].

The Messenger(p.b.u.h) said, "Whoever performs cupping on the 17th, 19th or 21st day (of the Islamic month) then it is a cure for every disease." [**Saheeh Sunan Abi Dawud (3861)**].

b) Is cupping from the Sunnah?

Above are just some of the authentic narrations which show that cupping is from the Sunnah of the Messenger (p.b.u.h) The Messenger (p.b.u.h) said, "Whoever revives a Sunnah from my Sunnah and the people practise it, s/he will have the same reward of those who practise it without their reward diminishing" [**Sunan ibn Maajah (209)**].

c) Cupping Is the Best of Remedies

Anas ibn Maalik (may Allah be pleased with him) reported that the Messenger (p.b.u.h) said, "Indeed the best of remedies you have is cupping" [**Saheeh al-Bukhaaree (5371)**].

Abu Hurairah (may Allaah be pleased with him) reported that the Messenger (p.b.u.h) said, "If there was something excellent to be used as a remedy then it is cupping." **[Saheeh Sunan abi Dawud (3857), Saheeh Sunan ibn Maajah (3476).**

d) The Angels Recommending Cupping

Abdullah ibn Abbas (may Allaah be pleased with him) reported that the Messenger (p.b.u.h) said, "I did not pass by an angel from the angels on the night journey except that they all said to me: Upon you is cupping, O Muhammad." [Saheeh Sunan ibn Maajah (3477)]. In the narration reported by Abdullah ibn Mas'ud (may Allah be pleased with him) the angels said, "Oh Muhammad, order your Ummah (nation) with cupping." [**Saheeh Sunan Tarmidhee (3479)**].

e) Cupping Is A Prevention?

Anas ibn Maalik (May Allah be pleased with him) reported that the Messenger (p.b.u.h) said, "Whoever wants to perform cupping then let him search for 17th, 19th and 21st and let none of you allow his blood to rage (boil) such that it kills him." [**Saheeh Sunan ibn Maajah (3486)**].

Anas ibn Maalik (may Allaah be pleased with him) reported that the Messenger (p.b.u.h) said, "When the weather becomes extremely hot, seek aid in cupping. Do not allow your blood to rage (boil) such that it kills you." [Reported by Hakim in his 'Mustadrak' and he authenticated it and Imam ad-Dhahabi agreed (4/212)].

f) In Cupping There Is A Cure And A blessing?

Abdullah ibn Abbas (May Allah be pleased with him) reported that the Messenger (p.b.u.h) said, "Healing is in three things: in the incision of the cupper, in drinking honey, and in cauterizing with fire, but I forbid my Ummah (nation) from cauterization (branding with fire)." **[Saheeh al-Bukhaaree (5681), Saheeh Sunan ibn Maajah (3491)]**.

Jaabir ibn Abdullah (may Allaah be pleased with him) reported that the Messenger (p.b.u.h) said, "Indeed in cupping there is a cure."**[Saheeh Muslim (5706)]**.

Ibn Umar (may Allaah be pleased with him) reported that the Messenger (p.b.u.h) said, "Cupping on an empty stomach is best. In it is a cure and a blessing..."**[Saheeh Sunan ibn Maajah (3487)]**.

'Alaa Ar-Reeq in arabic means to fast until after being treated with cupping. Once the treatment of cupping has been completed, one may eat and drink.

g) Cupping In Its Time Is A Cure For Every Disease?

Abu Hurairah (may Allaah be pleased with him) reported that the Messenger (p.b.u.h) said, "Whoever performs cupping on the 17th, 19th or 21st day (of the Islamic, lunar month) then it is a cure for every disease." **[Saheeh Sunan abi Dawud (3861)]**.

h) The Best Days for Cupping

The best days for cupping are the 17th, 19th and 21st of the Islamic month which coincide with Monday, Tuesday or Thursday. Anas ibn Maalik (may Allaah be pleased with him) reported that the Messenger (p.b.u.h) said, "Whoever wants to perform cupping then let him search for 17th, 19th and 21st day. [**Saheeh Sunan ibn Maajah (3486)**].

Ibn Umar (may Allaah be pleased with him) reported that the Messenger (p.b.u.h) said, "Cupping on an empty stomach* is best. In it is a cure and a blessing. It improves the intellect and the memory. So cup yourselves with the blessing of Allaah on Thursday. Perform cupping on Monday and Tuesday for it is the day that Allaah saved Ayoub from a trial. He was inflicted with the trial on Wednesday. You will not find leprosy except (by being cupped) on Wednesday or Wednesday night." [**Saheeh Sunan ibn Maajah (3487)**].

As for the Islamic day and night, the night enters before the day. So at sunset on Tuesday, Wednesday night comes in. Cupping is best performed during the daytime between the adhaan of fajr and the adhaan of maghrib because yawm in arabic means daytime. The Sunnah days for cupping every month are when the 17th or 19th or 21st of the lunar month coincide with a Monday, Tuesday or Thursday. These are the best and most beneficial days for cupping. If one is not able to be cupped on 17th, 19th or 21st (coinciding with Monday, Tuesday or Thursday) then any Monday, Tuesday or Thursday of the month.

l) Are you going to pump out all of my blood?

Relax! The blood that comes out is from the surface of the skin, it is not from the mainstream. If you are thinking your blood system only contains hemoglobin, platelets, plasma and white blood cells you are wrong, there are so many other junks that fly around in your body such as dead blood cells, blood clots, different toxins and pathogen. Different people's body give different responses, sometimes hardly anything comes out from a person's skin and that is a good thing. Because the cuts are very light the body heals the area very quick and automatically the blood stops coming out. We constantly analyze the patient if they are feeling well or not. Only in paradise you will be 100% pure and clean.

J) How long does it take to do hijama?

Depends how many cups you do, the standard five cups on the back takes approximately 45 mins.

K)How often should I do hijama?

It is totally up to you, some do it every month as a preventative medicine in the sunnah days, which is 17th, 19th and the 21st of the Islamic lunar calender. For non-veg.4 months d for vegetarian 6 months or even after a year depends. Hijama is a detoxification therapy, there are other detox programs that people follow for example, they may start to have more (organic) fruits and vegetables, antioxidant drinks, cut down on fatty unhealthy foods and so on.

L) I am pregnant can I do hijama?

No, you cannot do hijama if you are pregnant.

M) Can i do hijama if I had a miscarriage?

If you had a miscarriage recently we do not recommend hijama because after a miscarriage the body needs to rejuvenate itself, it can take close to 6 months to a year depending on the individual and how serious the miscarriage was, you must see your doctor before you try to conceive again. For sisters who had a miscarriage we strongly recommend to have a good nutrition diet with multivitamins everyday, believe me it will make a difference to your body. Avoid eating too much of carbs and spices e.g. rice, spice and red meat. Some sheikhs recommend for a woman after giving birth to wait at least 2 years before planning to get pregnant, because the body needs to fully recover and so on. You can try hijama after 6 months of your miscarriage (depending on what the doctor says and your situation), please make sure you are eating well and you do not need to fast before doing hijama. If you just ate we recommend for you to wait at least 2-3 hours before the hijama treatment.

N) What are the side effects of hijama?

NO SIDE EFFECTS ONLY EXTRA BENEFITS. However in some cases, possible side effects are feeling light headed, sick/nausea (especially in the morning on an empty stomach), fainting/blackout due to lack of energy and temporary bruising. These cases are very rare and only occur if the patient is very unwell.

Chapter 13

PATIENTS INFORMATION

PATIENTS INFORMATION:

What to expect?

Remember that Hijama is an easy yet very effective way of assisting your body to heal or prevent it from becoming imbalanced and consequently unwell. The therapist will show you a cup (there are different sizes of cups available, we will choose one that is appropriate for you) that will be placed either on the area/s of pain or on specific points of your body to promote healing or detoxification. We use disposable cups brand new, after using it on one patient we obviously get rid of it. We do not use glass cups with fire (also known as fire cupping) because No.1 accidents can happen and we do not want to end up burning our patients No.2 glass cups needs to be sterilized very well with good sterilizing tools, so just to be on the safe side we do not use glass cups. Everything we use is brand new from the pack.

Remember the cuts are very light scratches, and nothing is going in as the suction is always pulling out, this is a smart therapy, your skin filters/fights bacteria and other pathogens every day, so the chance of getting seriously infected is very low, especially when combined with the health and hygiene standard procedure.

Preparation before and after therapy:

Before:

The best advice is to fast; however, some people are unwell or feel very weak when fasting. It is better not to eat solid food for at least 2-3 hours before treatment so that the body is not occupied with digesting food. It is best to eat healthy food 24 hours before and after treatment. You are allowed to drink water.

After:

After the hijama session try to rest as some people feel very tired and need to relax or sleep. Others feel energised as they physically and psychologically feel refreshed; but do not exert yourself even if you feel like this. Do not underestimate the treatment and remember to respect the fact that your body needs rest in order to replenish and repair. Keep warm; do not allow the areas that have been treated to be exposed to the wind, water or cold. This also means no showers or baths for the next 2 hours. Try not to eat red meat and dairy products for the next 24 hours. This is because these items take up 40% of your body's energy to digest, and this energy is needed to rejuvenate your body after having the treatment.

FEW CLINICAL CASES PICTURES FOR DEMONSTRATION (Chapter 14)

FEW CLINICAL CASES PICTURES FOR DEMONSTRATION:

1. Timing and accu points of Cupping Therapy to Increase Fertility:

1. Around day 5 of the cycle until day 11 (stimulation)
2. Around day 12 of the cycle until day 16 (ovulation)
3. Around day 17 of the cycle until day 28 (luteal phase)

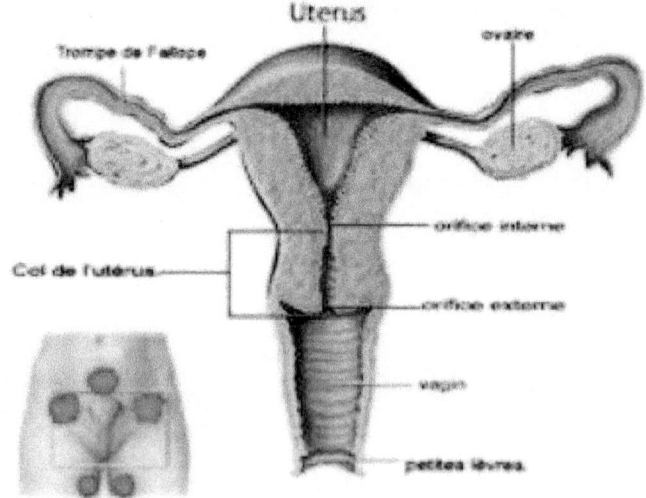

HIJAMA POINTS TO HEAL OVARIAN PROBLEMS, INFERTILITY INCLUDED...

2. Cupping therapy in Obsessive Compulsive Disorder (OCD) and Depression

Cupping/Hijamah (wet Cupping) therapy creates negative energy at minor incised key areas & points of the body using vacuumed cups. This process stimulates and boosts stagnant blood & other local congestion, mobilizes and extracts pathogenic & toxic substances.

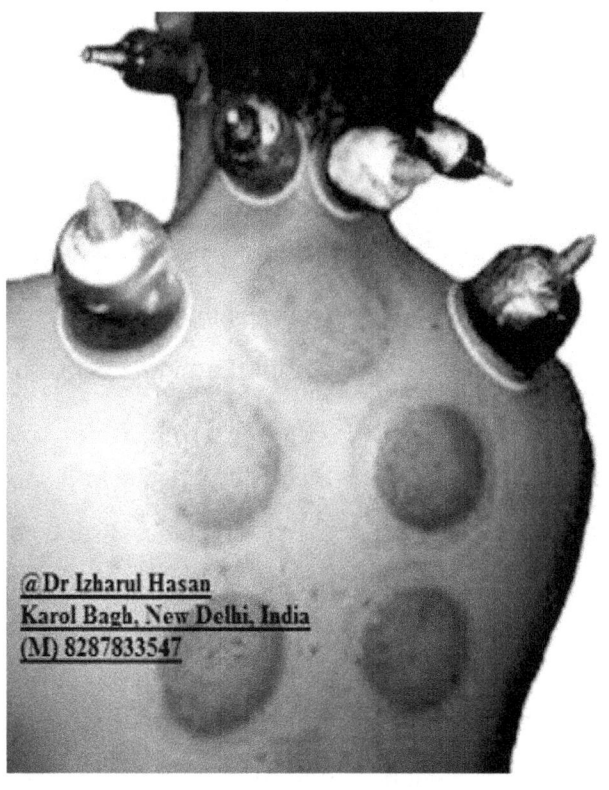

3. Cupping therapy on digestive system/liver/GB

The blood stagnation in the veins of the stomach and the intestines destroys their secretive and absorption functions and that will lead to severe bleeding, especially the vessels of the stomach, the intestines, the esophagus and the rectum, and blood clots in the legs and feet, hemorrhoids, and severe menstruation "in women", all of what mentioned above leads blood pressure to go down.

Cupping therapy activates the blood flow and consequently prevents blood from the in the digestive system. Therefore cupping prevents and treats all the above concerning problems.

Most patients have their complaints with hemorrhoids come to an END after performing cupping. The heightening blood pressure with a sluggish blood circulation leads to harm the biliary tracts and increases the density of the bile. Here cholesterol and bilirubin start to crystallize and that hinders the circulation of the arterial blood.

Whereas the compactness of the aged red corpuscles and their precipitation result in the impeded circulation in portal vein. Eventually, the tension of the portal vein heightens to push a part of the blood to the peripheral circulation round the liver through vessels anastomosis, consequently the spleen congests and enlarges and also does the venous vessels in the pancreas leading to its atrophy and its inability to do its functions. In fact, the cupping therapy is a prevention and cure for all these problems and saves us from lots of trouble.

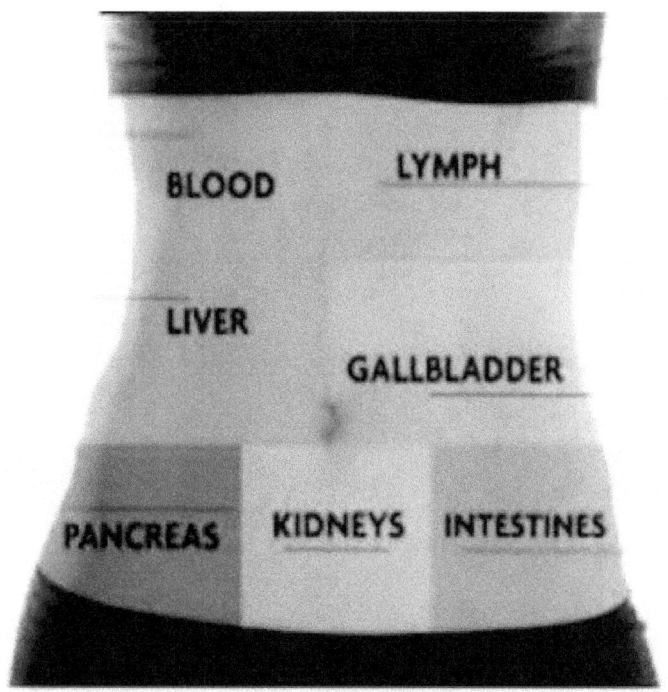

Cupping Therapy on Digestive system, Liver, GB, Pancreas & Intestines

4. Anxiety suffering patient treated successfully by cupping therapy

Anxiety is a normal human emotion that everyone experiences at times. Many people feel anxious, or nervous, when faced with a problem at work, before taking a test, or making an important decision. Anxiety disorders, however, are different. They can cause such distress that it interferes with a person's ability to lead a normal life. An anxiety disorder is a serious mental illness. For people with anxiety disorders, worry and fear are constant and overwhelming, and can be crippling.

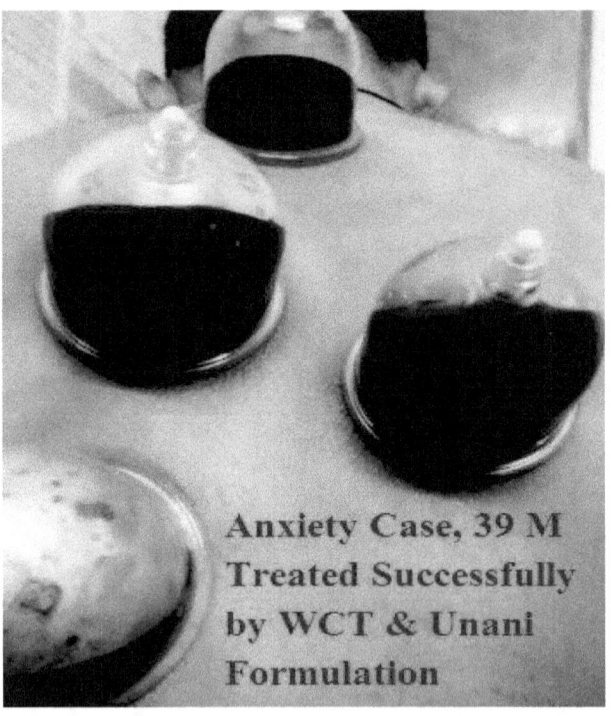

Anxiety Case, 39 M Treated Successfully by WCT & Unani Formulation

Anxiety disorders respond very well to treatment—and often in a relatively short amount of time. The specific treatment approach depends on the type of anxiety disorder and its severity. But in general, most anxiety disorders are treated with behavioral therapy, medication, or some combination of the two. In most cases complementary or alternative treatments especially in Unani system of medicine regimen cupping therapy have beneficial effects in such cases.

5. Dry Cupping therapy/whole body detoxification

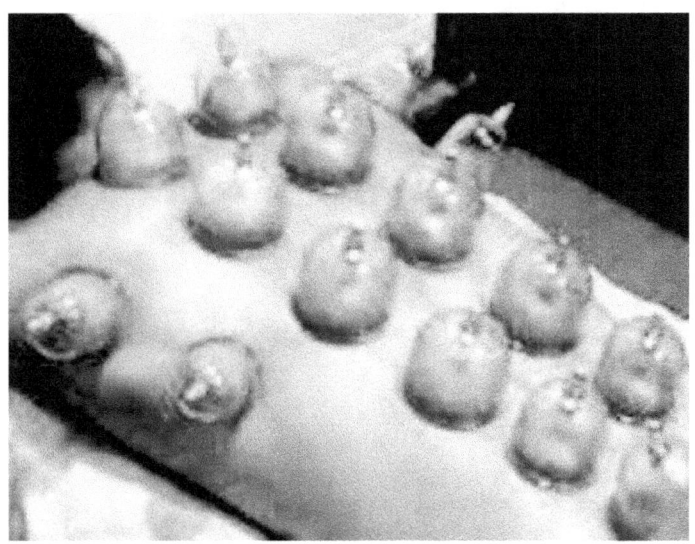

6. Cupping is an ancient method of treatment that has been used in the treatment and cure of a broad range of conditions; such as hypertension, rheumatic conditions ranging from arthritis, sciatica, back pain, migraine, anxiety and general physical and mental well-being. The aim of Cupping is to extract blood that is believed to be harmful from the body which in turn rids the body of potential harm from symptoms leading to a reduction in well-being. The Arabic name for Cupping Therapy is Al-Hejamah which means to reduce in size i.e. to return the body back to its natural state.

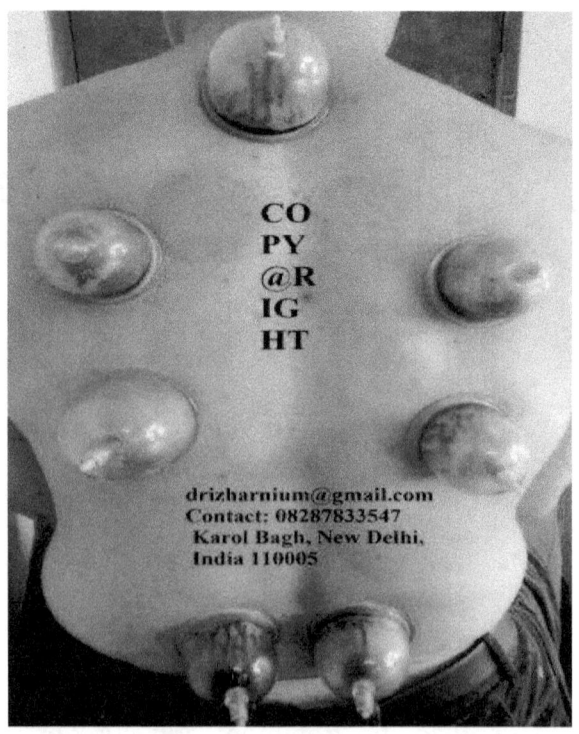

CO
PY
@R
IG
HT

drizharnium@gmail.com
Contact: 08287833547
Karol Bagh, New Delhi,
India 110005

7. Cupping therapy: an emergency for the management of angina / IHD patients.

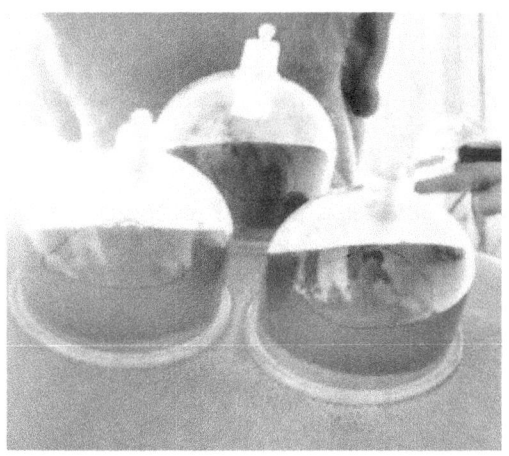

8. Migraine patient was treated successfully by applying cupping on these points

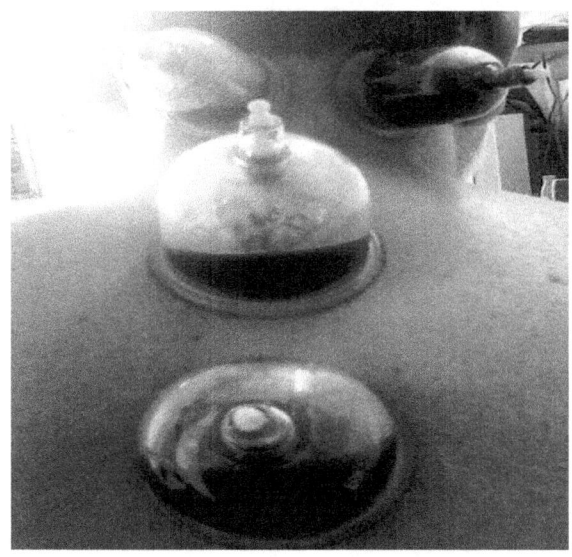

9. Cupping therapy in acute lower back pain

This case was determined according to standard Tibb and conventional clinical practice. That is, the researchers will assess the patients presenting signs and symptoms, with a clinical evaluation, possibly supported by the appropriate pathological testing, to confirm the diagnosis.

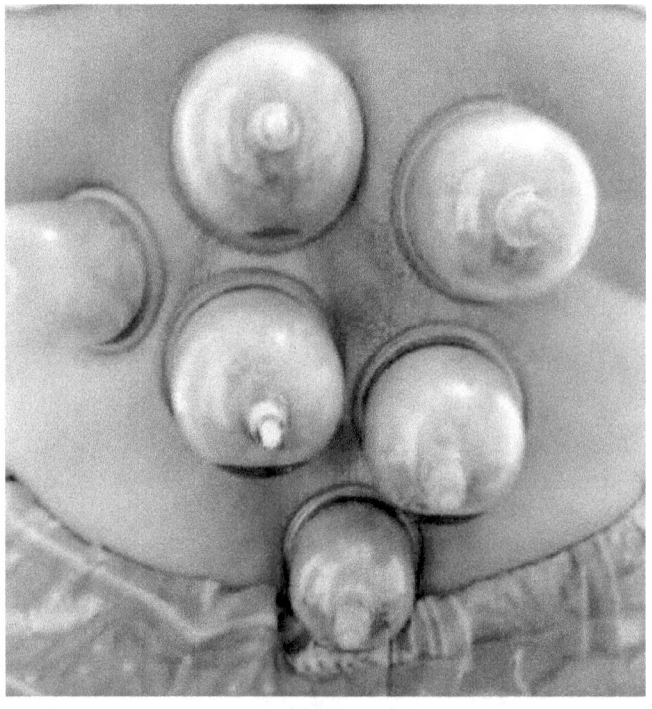

10. Cupping therapy in psoriasis suffering patient

Psoriasis is a common, chronic, recurrent disease of the skin characterized by rounded circumscribed dry erythematous , scaly patches of various size covered by multilayer greyish white or silver white scales which appear repeatedly on the erythema. The course of psoriasis is inconsistent, following an irregular chronic course marked by remissions andexacerbations of unpredictable onset and duration. Two of the chief features of psorisis are its tendency to recur and persist. This patient 39/M is suffering from nervous breakdown , psoriasis so on cupping therapy to get beneficial effects.

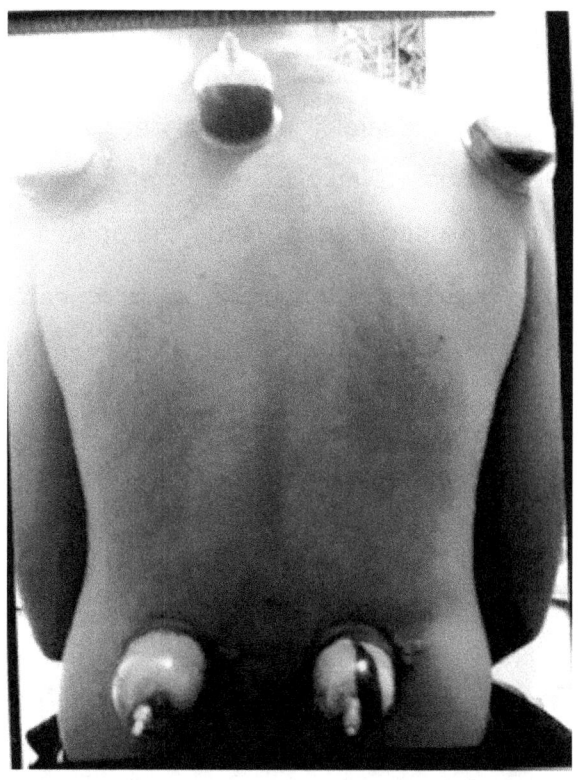

11. Cupping therapy in Myocardial Infarction, angina pectoris, Arrhythmias

Mohd Iqbal, 39 yrs/M, Delhi 06 H/o repeating attacks of angina pain

Cupping therapy has a therapeutic effect on cardiac and chest ailments including angina pectoris. cupping therapy not only quickly relieve the symptoms of acute angina pectoris, but also improve nitroglycerine's therapeutic effects. It is an efficient simple therapeutic method used for emergency and for regular angina treatment. Combination of conventional drug therapy and cupping therapy would considerably decrease the frequency and the required dosage of drug taking, thereby decreasing the unpleasant side effects of the drug therapy.

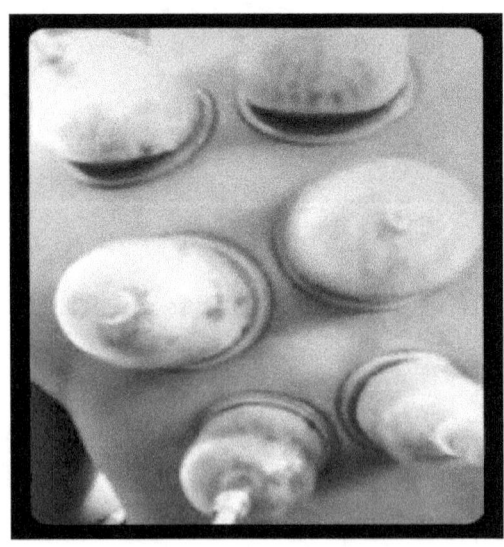

12. Cupping therapy done for immunity, respiratory and circulatory system

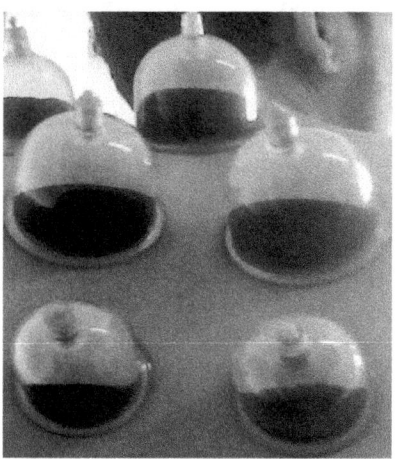

13. Cupping sites to improves circulation to the heart, reduce chest pain, cardiac spasm, and ischemia

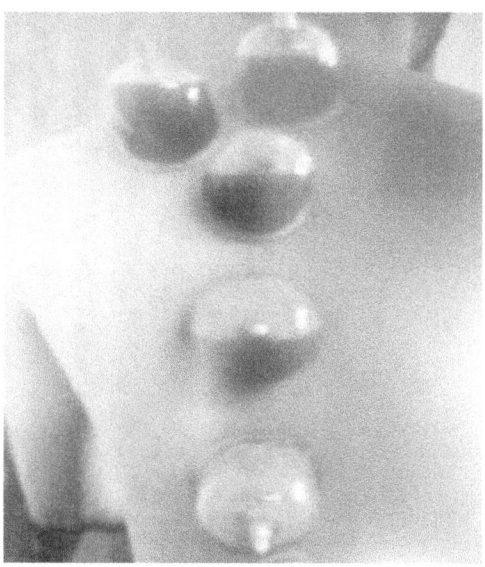

14. Durgadutt, age 59yrs, sex M, Diagnosed case of Type 2 Diabetes mellitus, HTN-ve, CAD/TMT +ve for stress induced ischemia.... cath and angio LAD mid to distal LAD d segment 70-75%, at mid segment 80-90%, mid RCA 100% filling..HBsAg/HCV/HIV -ve,...clinically managed through cupping therapy..before and after therapy RBS and subjective parameters are observing...therapy is done on the following points every 15 days...patient is clinically fitfor and continue on therapy...

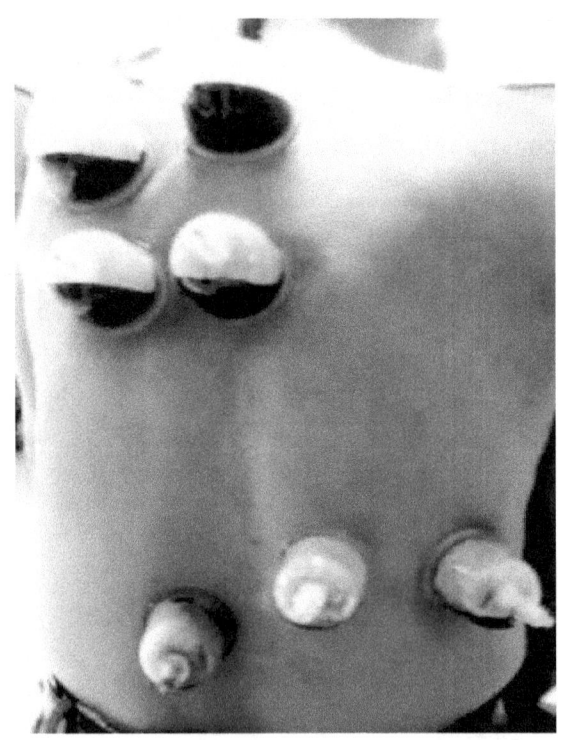

15. Wet cupping therapy

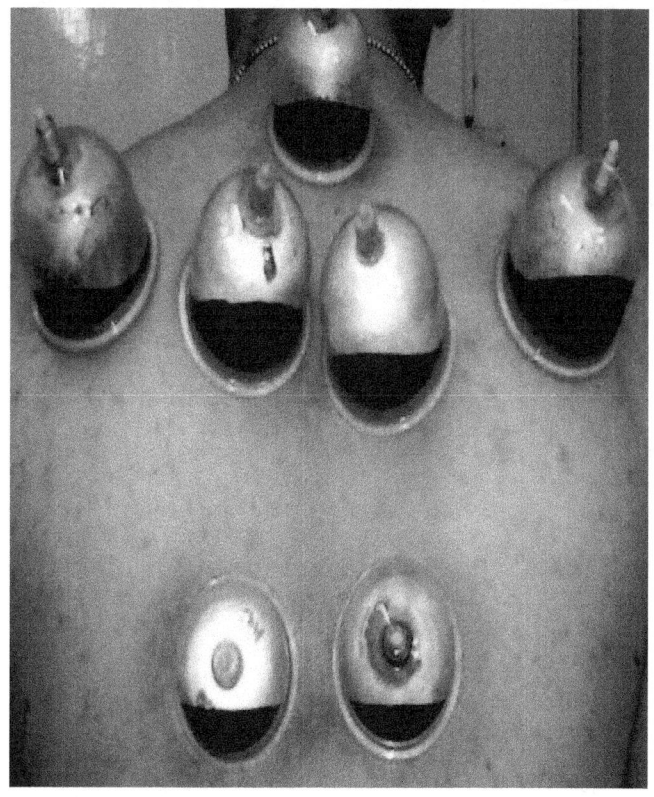

Chapter 15

SUMMARY AND REFERENCES

SUMMARY

Cupping is an ancient method of treatment that has been used in the treatment and cure of a broad range of conditions throughout the Eastern and Western cultures of the world. Conditions such as blood related disorders; haemophilia and hypertension for example, rheumatic conditions ranging from arthritis, sciatica, back pain and migraines through to psycho-social applications in the treatment of anxiety and general physical and mental well-being. Traditional theories advocate that the primary aim of Cupping is to extract blood that is believed to be harmful from the body which in turn rids the body of potential harm from symptoms leading to a reduction in well-being. To date there are no scientifically approved research trials anywhere in the world which investigated the impact of Cupping at a physiological level, although numerous small scale studies have been done promoting the benefits of Cupping for various diseases. In summary, al-Hijamah/cupping therapy is an authentic tradition of the Prophet (peace be upon him) that has been used throughout history. There is volume of anecdotal literature present however few scientific trials have investigated the effect of Cupping at various levels to the health. Evidence thus far points favourably for the use of Cupping as a treatment tool for a spectrum of medical ailments.

We pray to Allah to give us the ability to apply the knowledge he has given us in the best possible manner and that we continue to seek a better understanding in order to find cures for the illnesses he tests us with. And the best knowledge is with Allah, the Almighty.

REFERENCES:

1. Cui Jin and Zhang Guangqi, A survey of thirty years' clinical application of cupping, Journal of Traditional Chinese Medicine 1989; 9(3): 151-154.

2. Wu Jiashu, Observation of analgesic effect of acupuncturing dazhui point, Journal of Traditional Chinese Medicine 1989; 9(4): 240-242.

3. Ju Huadong, 30 cases of frozen shoulder treated by needling and cupping, International Journal of Clinical Acupuncture 1998; 9(3): 327-328.

4. Zhang Zhilong, Observation on therapeutic effects of blood-letting puncture with cupping in acute trigeminal neuralgia, Journal of Traditional Chinese Medicine 1997; 17(4): 272-274.

5. Cheng Xinnong, Chinese Acupuncture and Moxibustion, 1987 Foreign Languages Press, Beijing.

6. State Administration of Traditional Chinese Medicine and Pharmacy, Advanced Textbook on Traditional Chinese Medicine and Pharmacology, volume IV, 1997 New World Press, Beijing.

7. O'Conner J and Bensky D (translators), Acupuncture: A Comprehensive Text, 1981 Eastland Press, Seattle, WA.

8. Zhang Ruifu, Wu Xiufen, and Nissi Wang (compilers), Illustrated Dictionary of Chinese Acupuncture, 1986, Sheep's Publications, Hong Kong.

9. Academy of Traditional Chinese Medicine, An Outline of Chinese Acupuncture, 1975 Foreign Languages Press, Beijing.

10. Chen Decheng, Jiang Nawei, and Cong Xin, 47 cases of acne treated by prick-bloodletting plus cupping, Journal of Traditional Chinese Medicine 1993; 13(3): 185-186.

11. Wang Huaiping, Treatment of urticaria with cupping, Journal of Traditional Chinese Medicine 1993; 13(2): 105.

12. Li Jiang, A miraculous spinal pinching therapy, Journal of Traditional Chinese Medicine 1996; 16(3): 228-229.

13. Yin Ying, Blood-letting at a single point for treatment of acute diseases, Journal of

Traditional Chinese Medicine 1997; 17(3): 214-216.

14. Bayfield, S. (1839). A Practical Treatise on Cupping. Joseph Butler, London.

15. Brockbank, W. The Ancient Art of Cupping, The British Journal of Chinese Medicine, Vol1, No.21, Windhorse Press, London.

16. Cule, J (1980) A Doctor for the People: 2000 Years of General Practice in Britain. Update Books, London.

17. Cumston, CG (1987) The History of Medicine, Dorset Press, UK

18. Finerman, R. (1989) The Forgotten Healers: Women as Family Healers in an Andean Indian Community in CS

19. McClain (ed) Women as Healers: Cross Cultural Perspectives, Rutgers University Press, USA

20. Foucalt, M. (1976) The Birth of the Clinic, Tavistock, Great Britain.

21. Mettler, FA (1947) (ed) The History of Medicine, The Blakiston Co., Philadelphia.

22. Porter R. (1987), Disease Medicine and Society in England 1550-1860, Macmillan, London. Steven KH Aung (2002) Sexual Dysfunction: A Modern Medical Acupuncture Approach

23. Wan XW (2007) Clinical observation on treatment of cervical spondylosis with combined acupuncture and cupping therapies. Journal of Acupuncture and Tuina Science 5: 345-347.

24. Sommer AP, Pinheiro AL, Mester AR, Franke RP, Whelan HT (2001)Biostimulatory windows in low-intensity laser activation: lasers, scanners, and NASA's light-emitting diode array system. J Clin Laser Med Surg 19: 29-33.

25. Chirali IZ (1999) Traditional Chinese Medicine Cupping Therapy. In:The cupping procedure. Chirali IZ (1999) London: Churchill Livingstone 73-86.

26. Fu XY, Li Y, Yang JJ (2004) A survey of acupuncture for fibromyalgia

syndrome.Shanghai Journal of Acupuncture and Moxibustion 237: 46-48.

27. WARBURG O (1956) On the origin of cancer cells. Science 123: 309-314.

28. El Sayed SM, El-Magd RM, Shishido Y, Yorita K, Chung SP, et al. (2012)

29. D-Amino acid oxidase-induced oxidative stress, 3-bromopyruvate and citrate inhibit angiogenesis, exhibiting potent anticancer effects. J Bioenerg Biomembr 44: 513-523.

30. El Sayed SM, El-Magd RM, Shishido Y, Chung SP, Diem TH, et al. (2012) Bromopyruvate antagonizes effects of lactate and pyruvate, synergizes with citrate and exerts novel anti-glioma effects. J Bioenerg Biomembr 44: 61-79.

31. Nakano A, Tsuji D, Miki H, Cui Q, El Sayed SM, et al. (2011) Glycolysis inhibition inactivates ABC transporters to restore drug sensitivity in malignant cells. PLoS One 6: e27222.

32. El Sayed SM, Abou El-Magd RM, Shishido Y, Chung SP, Sakai T, et al. (2012) D-amino

acid oxidase gene therapy sensitizes glioma cells to the antiglycolytic effect of 3-bromopyruvate. Cancer Gene Ther 19: 1-18.

33. van Raam BJ, Sluiter W, de Wit E, Roos D, Verhoeven AJ, et al. (2008) Mitochondrial membrane potential in human neutrophils is maintained by complex III activity in the absence of supercomplex organisation. PLoS One 3e2013.

34. Robert K, Murray RK, Daryl K, Granner, Peter A, et al. (2003) Harper's illustrated biochemistry. 26th edition. Lange Medical Books/McGraw-Hill Medical Publishing Division 123.

35. El Sayed SM, Mahmoud, and Nabo MMH. Medical and Scientific Bases of Wet Cupping Therapy (Al-hijamah): in Light of Modern Medicine and Prophetic Medicine. Alternative and Integrative Medicine; V2, Issue 52013.

36. FACT, Focus on Alternative and Complementary Therapies, Abdullah Al Bedah,Mohamed Khalil, Ahmed Elolemy, Ibrahim Elsubai, Asim Khalil, Hijama (cupping):

a review of the evidence, Volume 16, Issue 1, pages 12-16, March 2011

37. FACT, Focus on Alternative and Complementary Therapies, Abdullah AlBedah, Mohamed Khalil, Ahmed Elolemy, Ibrahim Elsubai, Asim Khalil, Hijama (cupping): a review of the evidence, Volume 16, Issue 1, pages 12-16, March 2011

Book Details

Author: Izharul H.
Book Title: Encyclopedia of cupping therapy
Paperback: 182 pages
Publisher: First Edition: 2014
CSI Publishing Platform; 2nd edition (March, 2015)
Language: English
ISBN-10: **1508981507**
ISBN-13: **978-1508981503**
Product Dimensions: 6 x 9 inches

@2015 by publishing platform and author

Other Books of the author:

Essential Textbook of Preventive and Social Medicine

Humoral Pathology: Adjustment and Regulation

Essential Hand Book of Toxicology: For Medical Undergraduates

A Textbook of Regimenal Therapy: ...an unani speciality

Encyclopedia of Home Remedies to get Healthy Life

The Prime: MCQs for Post Graduation Unani Entrance Examination

The Premier, Previous Examination Papers Of MD Unani AMU Aligarh